Neurology Evidence

The Practice-Changing Studies

Kate T. Brizzi, MD
Instructor of Neurology
Department of Neurology
Massachusetts General Hospital
Harvard Medical School
Boston, Massachusetts

Ayush Batra, MD
Assistant Professor of Neurology
Ken & Ruth Davee Department of Neurology
Northwestern Memorial Hospital
Northwestern University Feinberg
   School of Medicine
Chicago, Illinois

Joel Salinas, MD, MBA, MSc
Instructor of Neurology
Department of Neurology
Massachusetts General Hospital
Harvard Medical School
Boston, Massachusetts

Nancy Wang, MD
Clinical Fellow
Pappas Center for Neuro-Oncology
Massachusetts General Hospital
Boston, Massachusetts

SERIES EDITORS

Emily L. Aaronson, MD
Erik L. Antonsen, MD, PhD
Arjun K. Venkatesh, MD, MBA, MHS

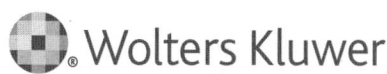

Wolters Kluwer

Philadelphia • Baltimore • New York • London
Buenos Aires • Hong Kong • Sydney • Tokyo

Acquisitions Editor: Chris Teja
Product Development Editor: Ashley Fischer
Editorial Coordinator: Lindsay Ries
Marketing Manager: Rachel Mante Leung
Production Project Manager: Bridgett Dougherty
Design Coordinator: Terry Mallon
Senior Manufacturing Coordinator: Beth Welsh
Prepress Vendor: S4Carlisle Publishing Services

9 8 7 6 5 4 3 2 1

Printed in China (or the United States of America)

Library of Congress Cataloging-in-Publication Data

Names: Batra, Ayush, editor. | Brizzi, Kate T., editor. | Salinas, Joel, editor. |
   Wang, Nancy, MD editor.
Title: Neurology evidence : the practice-changing studies / [edited by] Ayush Batra,
   Kate T. Brizzi, Joel Salinas, Nancy Wang.
Description: Philadelphia, PA : Wolters Kluwer, [2017] |
   Includes bibliographical references and index.
Identifiers: LCCN 2017016342 | ISBN 9781496348937
Subjects: | MESH: Nervous System Diseases—therapy | Clinical Trials as Topic
Classification: LCC RC346 | NLM WL 140 | DDC 616.8—dc23 LC record available at https://lccn.loc
   .gov/2017016342

LWW.com

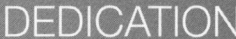

DEDICATION

To my parents, Dominic and Beverly Brizzi,
and my sister, Hannah Brizzi, who have provided
endless support.

Kate T. Brizzi, MD

To my parents, Arun and Dolly Batra, my brother,
Asheesh, and aunt, Suman, for their lifelong support;
and my wife, Nisha, for her encouragement to
help me succeed.

Ayush Batra, MD

To my parents, Norma and Armando Salinas,
my brother, Rainier Salinas, and my sister,
Scarlett Salinas, who have been a perpetual
source of genuine encouragement.

Joel Salinas, MD, MBA, MSc

To my parents, Hanyu Ni and Xu Wang, for being
my number one (and two) fans; my husband, David,
for his unwavering support; and my dear Everett for
inspiring me to be my best.

Nancy Wang, MD

CONTRIBUTORS

Anna M. Bank, MD
Resident Physician
Partners Neurology Residency
Brigham and Women's Hospital
Massachusetts General Hospital
Harvard Medical School
Boston, Massachusetts

Michael P. Bowley, MD, PhD
Instructor of Neurology
Harvard Medical School
Assistant in Neurology
Massachusetts General Hospital
Boston, Massachusetts

Sheena Chew, MD
Resident Physician
Partners Neurology Residency
Brigham and Women's Hospital
Massachusetts General Hospital
Harvard Medical School
Boston, Massachusetts

Christopher Doughty, MD
Resident Physician
Partners Neurology Residency
Brigham and Women's Hospital
Massachusetts General Hospital
Harvard Medical School
Boston, Massachusetts

Brian L. Edlow, MD
Assistant Professor of Neurology
Massachusetts General Hospital
Harvard Medical School
Boston, Massachusetts

Mark R. Etherton, MD, PhD
Vascular Neurology Fellow
Department of Neurology
Massachusetts General Hospital
Harvard Medical School
Boston, Massachusetts

Steven K. Feske, MD
Associate Professor of Neurology
Harvard Medical School
Chief of Cerebrovascular Division
Department of Neurology
Brigham and Women's Hospital
Harvard Medical School
Boston, Massachusetts

Maya Srikanth Graham, MD PhD
Resident Physician
Partners Neurology Residency
Brigham and Women's Hospital
Massachusetts General Hospital
Harvard Medical School
Boston, Massachusetts

Steven M. Greenberg, MD, PhD
Professor of Neurology
Massachusetts General Hospital
Harvard Medical School
Boston, Massachusetts

Todd Herrington, MD, PhD
Instructor in Neurology
Harvard Medical School
Assistant in Neurology
Massachusetts General Hospital
Boston, Massachusetts

Tamara B. Kaplan, MD
Instructor of Neurology
Department of Neurology
Partners MS Center
Brigham and Women's Hospital
Harvard Medical School
Boston, Massachusetts

David J. Lin, MD
Resident Physician
Partners Neurology Residency
Brigham and Women's Hospital
Massachusetts General Hospital
Harvard Medical School
Boston, Massachusetts

Jennifer L. Lyons, MD
Assistant Professor of Neurology
Brigham and Women's Hospital
Harvard Medical School
Boston, Massachusetts

Scott M. McGinnis, MD
Assistant Professor of Neurology
Brigham and Women's Hospital
Harvard Medical School
Boston, Massachusetts

Emer McGrath, MB, BCh, PhD, MRCP
Resident Physician
Partners Neurology Residency
Brigham and Women's Hospital
Massachusetts General Hospital
Harvard Medical School
Boston, Massachusetts

Kathleen E. McKee, MD
Resident Physician
Partners Neurology Residency
Brigham and Women's Hospital
Massachusetts General Hospital
Harvard Medical School
Boston, Massachusetts

Saad Mir, MD
Vascular Neurology Fellow
Department of Neurology
New York Presbyterian Hospital
Weill Cornell Medical Center
New York, New York

William Mullally, MD
Associate Chief of Clinical Neurology
Brigham and Women's Hospital
Assistant Professor of Neurology
Harvard Medical School
Boston, Massachusetts

Patricia L. Musolino, MD, PhD
Assistant Professor of Neurology
Critical Care and Vascular Neurology
Center for Genomic Medicine
Massachusetts General Hospital
Harvard Medical School
Boston, Massachusetts

Abby L. Olsen, MD, PhD
Resident Physician
Partners Neurology Residency
Brigham and Women's Hospital
Massachusetts General Hospital
Harvard Medical School
Boston, Massachusetts

Mikael L. Rinne, MD, PhD
Instructor in Neurology
Center for Neuro-Oncology
Dana-Farber/Brigham and Women's
  Cancer Center
Harvard Medical School
Boston, Massachusetts

Daniel B. Rubin, MD, PhD
Resident Physician
Partners Neurology Residency
Brigham and Women's Hospital
Massachusetts General Hospital
Harvard Medical School
Boston, Massachusetts

Altaf Saadi, MD
Resident Physician
Partners Neurology Residency
Brigham and Women's Hospital
Massachusetts General Hospital
Harvard Medical School
Boston, Massachusetts

James Stankiewicz, MD
Clinical Director
Partners Multiple Sclerosis Center
Brigham and Women's Hospital
Assistant Professor of Neurology
Harvard Medical School
Boston, Massachusetts

Jesse M. Thon, MD
Resident Physician
Partners Neurology Residency
Brigham and Women's Hospital
Massachusetts General Hospital
Harvard Medical School
Boston, Massachusetts

Henrikas Vaitkevicius, MD
Instructor of Neurology
Neurocritical Care
Brigham and Women's Hospital
Harvard Medical School
Boston, Massachusetts

Nagagopal Venna, MD, MRCPI, MRCPUK
Associate Professor of Neurology
Chief of Comprehensive Neurology Division
Director of Advanced General and
    Autoimmune Neurology Fellowship
Massachusetts General Hospital
Harvard Medical School
Boston, Massachusetts

Melissa A. Walker, MD, PhD
Instructor of Neurology
Department of Neurology
Massachusetts General Hospital
Harvard Medical School
Boston, Massachusetts

M. Brandon Westover, MD, PhD
Assistant Professor of Neurology
Neurology Department, Epilepsy Service
Massachusetts General Hospital
Harvard Medical School
Boston, Massachusetts

Let us witness with great relief the effect of logic and proof on modern neurology. Whereas, in the past there were authoritative but annoying pronouncements from senior (and not so senior) clinicians about the value of one therapy or another, about one approach to a disease or another, we can finally be guided by some actual evidence. The turn of events that brought clinical trials to bear on neurological practice starting in the late 1980s was turbulent, as acolytes of various schools adhered to advice garnered from the accumulated wisdom of their mentors, at times bordering on cultism. Clinical trials were late to come to neurology, well after cardiology, for example, had capitulated to the results of increasingly well-designed studies.

Early trials in neurology were marred by what would now be considered poor design, but indispensable lessons were learned about powering, prespecified primary and secondary outcomes, correction for multiple comparisons, imputation for missing data, noninferiority testing, subgroup analysis, and appropriate statistical methods. We still are struggling with some of these, but there is equivalent importance to proof that a new treatment proves to be useful, or is shown not to be useful, or even harmful, and can then be virtually discarded.

This is not to say that valuable things have not been lost in the deluge of trials. Regarding clinical trials, C. Miller Fisher—whose guidance on stroke therapy derived from carefully recorded observation was dictum for decades—said in my presence, "There ain't no more than one average Englishman," and Lou Caplan's partial but incisive rejoinder to trials, "What's wrong with Mrs. Jones," reminds us that we need to avoid the same slavish devotion to trial results that we had in the past to anecdotal evidence. (By the way, the methods employed by Fisher were only deceptively anecdotal, and he turned out to be right about most stroke treatments he promoted.) It is common knowledge that large trials give credibility to outcomes in groups of patients, not necessarily to individual patients. But that may not be the point, because a clinician confronted by a single patient still needs to know the odds of helping or hurting with each course of action.

That is the incredible value of this book. We finally have a reasoned compendium of trials that guide the treatment of neurological disease and a decoding of the creative acronyms that name the trials. The strengths and weaknesses of both seminal and less-noticed studies are analyzed, and a readable commentary is offered by both a senior and junior neurologist to front-line clinicians at all levels. These studies and their narratives are vital to practice, both in academics and in the community. Indeed, knowledge of the results and, more importantly, the strengths and weaknesses of each study should become the new roundsmanship in teaching hospitals and a source of confidence for all practitioners. So, I say, it's about time and well done. I will be using this resource constantly and look forward to its inevitable updating.

Allan H. Ropper, MD

With the steady increase of diagnostic and therapeutic interventions in neurology, making the treatment decision that is in the best interest of the patient, balanced with public health interest at large, is one of the pivotal concerns a clinical neurologist faces with each patient interaction. The most historical and intuitive approach is to fall back on the practice habits deliberately and subconsciously ingrained throughout the course of medical training. The presumed expectation is that what was done before continues to be the best course of action today. Much has been learned over the last several decades through the steadfast dedication of clinician-investigators and the generous commitment of study participants. Harnessing the insights gained from positive and negative trials has proven to be critical in the ongoing improvement of clinical outcomes for patients suffering from neurological disease.

The path to treatments that are safe, timely, effective, efficient, equitable, and patient-centered—as defined by the Institute of Medicine—is rarely clear and linear. Because of the meandering course toward the discovery and interpretation of evidence that can lead to concrete changes in clinical practice, a compendium of the studies that have the greatest impact on how neurologists care for patients is needed. *Neurology Evidence* was inspired by this need to serve as a reference for both trainees beginning to learn their craft and experienced neurologists seeking to review how decades of research have guided us to the present.

To accomplish the colossal task of selecting, summarizing, and evaluating the most relevant papers to the practice of neurology today, the editors worked alongside many of the most accomplished and renowned neurologists across each subspecialty field to select studies for each clinical topic. There are far too many superb clinical trials and studies to include all. Thus, the list was narrowed with care to the top 100 papers that had the most significant impact on changing clinical practice—in other words, what differentiates the contemporary neurologists from the historical giants who laid the foundation for modern neurology. Once the papers were selected, each study was interpreted by residents and fellows passionate about the particular topic. The study summaries, with the guidance of senior authors, focus on maximizing relevance of information provided, engaging readers through questions and answers, and shedding light on future directions in each area of study. It is the editors' sincere hope that *Neurology Evidence* will help to make the vast body of literature that exists in neurology more accessible to neurologists and students at all levels. In doing so, we hope to inspire greater clarity and confidence in the valuable care we deliver to neurological patients and, if we are lucky, inspire the next generation of practice-changing studies in neurology.

ACKNOWLEDGMENTS

The editors are deeply grateful for the support and guidance of many colleagues and friends who helped bring this book to fruition. We would also like to thank the Partners Neurology residents, fellows, and faculty who contributed to the review and interpretation of each of the studies for their time and commitment. Additionally, we extend a special thank you to Dr. Allan H. Ropper for encouraging the creation of this book and for lending his rich experience and insight.

CONTENTS

SECTION 1: ISCHEMIC STROKE
Authors: Steven K. Feske, Mark R. Etherton, Jesse M. Thon

SECTION 2: CEREBRAL HEMORRHAGE
Authors: Steven M. Greenberg, David J. Lin, Saad Mir

SECTION 3: TRAUMATIC BRAIN INJURY
Authors: Brian L. Edlow, Daniel B. Rubin

SECTION 4: NEUROLOGIC INTENSIVE CARE
Authors: Henrikas Vaitkevicius, David J. Lin

SECTION 5: NEUROINFECTIOUS DISEASES
Authors: Jennifer L. Lyons, Altaf Saadi

SECTION 6: NEURO-ONCOLOGY
Authors: Mikael L. Rinne, Maya Srikanth Graham

SECTION 7: NEUROMUSCULAR
Authors: Michael P. Bowley, Kathleen E. McKee

SECTION 8: MOVEMENT DISORDERS
Authors: Todd Herrington, Abby L. Olsen

SECTION 9: MULTIPLE SCLEROSIS
Authors: James Stankiewicz, Tamara B. Kaplan

SECTION 10: AUTOIMMUNE NEUROLOGY
Authors: Nagagopal Venna, Christopher Doughty

SECTION 11: EPILEPSY
Authors: M. Brandon Westover, Anna M. Bank

SECTION 12: HEADACHE AND PAIN
Authors: William Mullally, Sheena Chew

SECTION 13: COGNITIVE NEUROLOGY
Authors: Scott M. McGinnis, Emer McGrath

SECTION 14: PEDIATRIC NEUROLOGY
Authors: Patricia L. Musolino, Melissa A. Walker

SECTION 1

ISCHEMIC STROKE

Steven K. Feske ■ Mark R. Etherton ■ Jesse M. Thon

1. Intravenous tPA for Acute Ischemic Stroke
2. Aspirin for Secondary Stroke Prevention
3. Mechanical Thrombectomy for Large Vessel Occlusion
4. Harm from Stenting of Symptomatic Intracranial Arterial Stenoses
5. Warfarin for Atrial Fibrillation
6. Novel Oral Anticoagulants for Stroke Prevention in Nonvalvular Atrial Fibrillation
7. Intense Low-Density Lipoprotein Cholesterol Reduction for Stroke Prevention
8. Marginal Benefit from Device Closure of Patent Foramen Ovale
9. Early Decompressive Surgery in Malignant Infarction of the Middle Cerebral Artery
10. Carotid Endarterectomy for Stroke Prevention in Internal Carotid Artery Stenosis
11. Carotid Artery Stenting vs. Carotid Endarterectomy for Symptomatic and Asymptomatic Carotid Artery Stenosis
12. Warfarin and Aspirin in Patients with Heart Failure and Sinus Rhythm
13. Short-Term Dual Antiplatelet Therapy for Stroke Prevention after TIA or Minor Stroke
14. Aspirin over Warfarin for Symptomatic Intracranial Stenosis
15. Lack of Benefit from Long-Term Dual Antiplatelet Therapy for Secondary Stroke Prevention
16. Fluoxetine for Motor Recovery after Acute Ischemic Stroke
17. Carotid Endarterectomy for Asymptomatic Carotid Artery Stenosis
18. Extended Monitoring for Paroxysmal Atrial Fibrillation
19. The National Institutes of Health Stroke Scale

CHAPTER 1

INTRAVENOUS tPA FOR ACUTE ISCHEMIC STROKE

Tissue Plasminogen Activator for Acute Ischemic Stroke

The National Institute of Neurological Disorders and Stroke rt-PA Study Group. *NEJM*. 1995;333(24):1581–1587

BACKGROUND

At the time of this study, there was no direct treatment to improve neurologic outcomes in acute ischemic stroke. Because the great majority of ischemic strokes are known to be the result of thrombotic occlusions, the authors speculated that early thrombolytic recanalization could reduce the degree of injury. Two smaller, open-label studies of intravenous (IV) tPA had suggested that early treatment within 180 minutes of stroke onset could reduce the risk of intracranial hemorrhage and maximize neurologic recovery.

OBJECTIVES

To assess the risks and benefits of IV tPA administered for treatment of acute ischemic stroke.

METHODS

Randomized, placebo-controlled trial conducted in two parts at eight centers across the United States from 1991 to 1994.

Patients

624 patients with acute ischemic stroke treated within 90 minutes (302 patients) or 180 minutes (322 patients) from stroke onset with defined time of onset, measurable deficit on National Institutes of Health stroke scale (NIHSS), and computed tomographic (CT) scan of the brain without evidence of intracranial hemorrhage. Average age was 66 to 69 years, and median NIHSS score was 14 to 15 in each group. Exclusion criteria included no stroke in preceding 3 months, major surgery within 14 days, systolic blood pressure >185 mm Hg, rapidly improving symptoms, or gastrointestinal hemorrhage within previous 21 days.

Interventions

Patients received placebo or alteplase at a dose of 0.9 mg/kg body weight (maximum 90 mg); 10% of alteplase dose administered as bolus followed by remaining 90% infused over 60 minutes.

Outcomes

Primary outcome for Part 1 was defined as complete resolution of neurologic deficit or improvement in NIHSS by 4 or more points 24 hours after stroke onset. The primary outcome in Part 2 was minimal or no deficit 3 months after treatment as assessed by a composite of four outcome measures (the Wald test), including the modified Rankin scale (mRS), Barthel index, Glasgow outcome scale, and NIHSS. The secondary outcomes were intention-to-treat analyses for outcomes at 3 months in Part 1 and NIHSS measurement at 24 hours in Part 2.

KEY RESULTS

- In Part 1, there was no significant difference in primary outcome of complete resolution of neurologic deficits at 24 hours (67% vs. 57%, RR = 1.2, 95% CI = 0.9–1.6, $p = 0.21$). (However, in Part 2 and in the analysis of the combined patients from Parts 1 and 2, there was a significant benefit at 24 hours for those treated within 90 minutes.)
- In Part 2, there was a significant benefit in the tPA group for the primary outcome combining three functional measures and the NIHSS at 3 months (OR = 1.7, 95% CI = 1.2–2.6, $p = 0.008$). (A similar significant benefit at 3 months was found in Part 1 and in the combined analysis.)
- There was a 12% absolute increase at 3 months in the number of patients with minimal or no disability (Barthel index score > 95) in the tPA group.
- Symptomatic intracerebral hemorrhage occurred in 6.4% of tPA group and only 0.6% of placebo group ($p < 0.001$).

STUDY CONCLUSIONS

Despite an increased incidence of intracerebral hemorrhage, IV tPA administered within 3 hours of acute ischemic stroke improves clinical outcomes at 3 months.

COMMENTARY

This study validated the use of IV tPA for the treatment of acute ischemic stroke within 180 minutes of stroke onset as a relatively safe and effective therapy. On subgroup analysis, the authors demonstrated that tPA administered within 90 minutes of stroke significantly increases the number of participants with complete resolution of neurologic symptoms (55% vs. 42%, $p = 0.02$). Treatment with tPA increased the odds of a more favorable outcome irrespective of stroke subtype. This study represents the first positive placebo-controlled trial for a direct medical therapy for acute ischemic stroke, which revolutionized the management of acute ischemic stroke by transforming the emphasis of medical care to the rapid evaluation for eligibility for IV tPA and for its prompt administration.

Question

Is IV tPA safe and effective for acute ischemic stroke?

Answer

Yes, IV tPA represents the first direct medical treatment for acute ischemic stroke that improves functional outcomes.

CHAPTER 2

ASPIRIN FOR SECONDARY STROKE PREVENTION

Collaborative Overview of Randomised Trials of Antiplatelet Therapy—I: Prevention of Death, Myocardial Infarction, and Stroke by Prolonged Antiplatelet Therapy in Various Categories of Patients

Antiplatelet Trialists' Collaboration. *BMJ.* 1994;308:81–106

BACKGROUND

Antiplatelet therapy reduces the risk of vascular death and nonfatal myocardial infarction (MI) and stroke in patients with unstable angina. At the time of this collaboration, however, there was uncertainty regarding a benefit for prolonged antiplatelet therapy in high-risk subpopulations, including patients with prior transient ischemic attacks (TIAs) or ischemic strokes. In a select population of patients, antiplatelet therapy had been demonstrated to be efficacious; however, the applicability to other demographics and the risk/benefit of long-term antiplatelet therapy among subjects at lower risk of occlusive vascular disease was unclear.

OBJECTIVES

To evaluate the effects of antiplatelet therapy on nonfatal strokes, vascular deaths, or nonfatal MI in various patient populations.

METHODS

Meta-analysis of 257 eligible randomized trials on antiplatelet therapy; analyzed until March 1990.

Patients

118,958 patients were subdivided into "high risk" (those with evidence of prior vascular disease, approximately 70,000 patients) and "low risk" (no prior evidence of vascular disease, approximately 30,000 patients).

Interventions

Antiplatelet regimens included various doses and durations of aspirin, aspirin combined with dipyridamole, dipyridamole, or sulphinpyrazone.

Outcomes

Effect of antiplatelet therapy on vascular events defined as nonfatal MI, nonfatal strokes, or vascular death was the primary outcome measure. Transient ischemic attacks were excluded.

KEY RESULTS

- Composite primary outcome of vascular event was reduced by 25% in "high-risk" groups with antiplatelet therapy vs. control: acute MI 10% vs. 14%, prior MI 13% vs. 17%, prior stroke or transient ischemic attack (TIA) 18% vs. 22% ($p < 0.0001$).

- The "low-risk" group had benefit for antiplatelet therapy in reduction of nonfatal MI (1.5% vs. 2.0%, $p < 0.0005$) and no decrease in nonfatal strokes (1.1% vs. 0.9%, nonsignificant).
- There was no significant difference in protective effects of high-dose (>500 mg) vs. medium-dose (75 to 325 mg) aspirin for vascular events.

STUDY CONCLUSIONS

In patients at high risk of occlusive vascular disease, antiplatelet therapy offers protection against nonfatal stroke, MI, and death.

COMMENTARY

The Antiplatelet Trialists' Collaboration study was done to evaluate the broad applicability and safety of antiplatelet therapy for the prevention of occlusive vascular disease. The importance of this analysis was predicated on its massive scope and number of trials analyzed. The dramatic benefit of antiplatelet therapy for reductions in vascular events was statistically significant for men and women separately, hypertensive and normotensive patients, and diabetic and nondiabetic patients. The series of papers by the Antiplatelet Trialists' Collaboration altered clinical practice by strongly emphasizing the role of antiplatelet therapy for prevention of recurrent vascular events including stroke.

Question

Does antiplatelet therapy in patients at high risk of vascular occlusive disease reduce recurrent vascular events?

Answer

Yes, in patients with documented atherosclerosis, prolonged antiplatelet therapy reduces recurrent vascular events.

CHAPTER 3

MECHANICAL THROMBECTOMY FOR LARGE VESSEL OCCLUSION

A Randomized Trial of Intraarterial Treatment for Acute Ischemic Stroke

Berkhemer OA, Fransen PSS, Beumer D, et al. *NEJM*. 2015;372:11–20

BACKGROUND

Large artery occlusions of the anterior circulation represent a common and severely debilitating form of ischemic stroke. In addition, IV tPA has limited ability to recanalize such proximal occlusions of the intracranial arteries. Prior to the Multicenter Randomized Clinical Trial of Endovascular Treatment for Acute Ischemic Stroke in the Netherlands (MR CLEAN), three randomized controlled trials (RCTs) using intraarterial (IA) therapies (MR RESCUE, IMS III, and SYNTHESIS Expansion) had failed to show a benefit on functional outcomes. In the design of MR CLEAN, the authors speculated that improved patient selection and newer endovascular devices would improve outcomes.

OBJECTIVES

To assess whether IA treatment added to IV tPA improves functional outcomes in patients with ischemic strokes secondary to occlusion of the proximal anterior circulation.

METHODS

Multicenter, randomized blinded end-point evaluation trial conducted at 16 centers in the Netherlands between December 2010 and March 2014.

Patients

500 patients with acute ischemic stroke due to occlusion of a proximal intracranial artery in the anterior circulation (distal ICA, M1/M2, or A1/A2), established by computed tomographic angiography (CTA), magnetic resonance angiography (MRA), or digital subtraction angiography, were randomized. Notable inclusion criteria included age >18 years, NIHSS ≥ 2, and possibility of treatment within 6 hours of symptom onset. Median NIHSS was 17 to 18 and median alberta stroke program early CT score (ASPECTS) was 9 in each group.

Interventions

IA treatment plus usual care (IV tPA) vs. usual care alone. In the intervention group, IA treatment consisted of delivery of a thrombolytic agent, mechanical thrombectomy, or both.

Outcomes

Primary outcome was the overall distribution of scores on mRS at 90 days. Secondary outcomes included dichotomized mRS scores at 90 days, NIHSS at 24 hours and 5 to 7 days, 90-day Barthel index score, and EuroQol Group five dimensions self-report questionnaire (EQ-5D quality of life assessment).

KEY RESULTS

- Median mRS at 90 days was improved in the IA group (3 vs. 4, aOR = 1.67, 95% CI = 1.21–2.30).
- mRS ≤ 2 improved in the IA group (32.6% vs. 19.1%, aOR = 2.16, 95% CI = 1.39–3.38).
- NIHSS at 5 to 7 days was reduced in the IA group (8 vs. 14, beta = 2.9, 95% CI = 1.5–4.3).
- Good reperfusion (modified TICI 2b or 3) was achieved in 58.7% of the IA group.
- Retrievable stents were used in 82% of the IA group.

STUDY CONCLUSIONS

In patients with acute ischemic stroke secondary to proximal occlusion of an anterior circulation artery, IA treatment within 6 hours from stroke onset improves functional outcomes.

COMMENTARY

MR CLEAN showed that IA treatment is safe and effective for the management of ischemic stroke secondary to proximal occlusion of the anterior circulation. In contrast to prior studies (IMS III, SYNTHESIS Expansion, and MR RESCUE), MR CLEAN demonstrated that early intervention with second-generation mechanical thrombectomy devices in documented occlusions of the proximal anterior circulation significantly improved functional outcomes at 90 days. Later in 2015, four additional studies (ESCAPE in Canada, EXTEND-IA in Australia, SWIFT PRIME in the United States and Europe, and REVASCAT in Spain), which were stopped prematurely after MR CLEAN was reported, further supported these findings. In all of these studies, patients had documented large artery occlusions (in contrast to prior studies) and some used additional imaging modalities to optimize the identification of patients most likely to benefit (e.g., infarct core size by ASPECTS, perfusion imaging, or collateral grade). This study revolutionized the management of acute ischemic stroke secondary to proximal occlusions of the anterior circulation.

Question

Is IA treatment safe and effective for patients with acute ischemic stroke secondary to proximal occlusion of the anterior circulation?

Answer

Yes, IA treatment administered within 6 hours of stroke onset is safe and effective in this patient population.

CHAPTER 4

HARM FROM STENTING OF SYMPTOMATIC INTRACRANIAL ARTERIAL STENOSES

Stenting versus Aggressive Medical Therapy for Intracranial Arterial Stenoses

Chimowitz MI, Lynn MJ, Derdeyn CP, et al; SAMMPRIS Trial Investigators. *NEJM*. 2011;365:993–1003

BACKGROUND

Atherosclerotic intracranial arterial stenosis represents a common cause of ischemic stroke. Patients with severe stenosis are at a high risk of recurrent stroke in the territory supplied by the stenotic artery. Percutaneous transluminal angioplasty and stenting (PTAS) of intracranial arterial stenosis was increasingly used to prevent recurrent strokes. At the time of this study, there was uncertainty regarding the optimal treatment of intracranial arterial stenosis with aggressive medical therapy alone vs. in combination with PTAS.

OBJECTIVES

To compare maximum medical therapy with PTAS for secondary ischemic stroke prevention in recently symptomatic patients with intracranial arterial stenosis.

METHODS

Prospective, randomized study at 50 centers across the United States between 2008 and 2011.

Patients

451 patients who experienced a TIA or nondisabling stroke secondary to an angiographically confirmed stenosis of 70% to 90% within 30 days before enrollment were randomized. There was no significant difference in the degree of stenosis or location of the qualifying artery between groups.

Interventions

Aggressive medical management (MM) consisted of aspirin 325 mg and clopidogrel 75 mg daily for 90 days after enrollment, systolic blood pressure < 140 mm Hg, and low-density lipoprotein (LDL) < 70 mg/dL. The PTAS group received aggressive MM and underwent placement of a Wingspan stent across the lesion.

Outcomes

Primary end points were any stroke or death within 30 days after enrollment or revascularization and ischemic stroke in territory of qualifying artery beyond 30 days. Secondary outcomes included any stroke or death, MI, or major hemorrhage.

KEY RESULTS

- Enrollment was stopped early because of an excess of stroke and death in the PTAS group.

- Primary end point of stroke or death within 30 days after enrollment or revascularization for qualifying artery beyond 30 days: 20.5% PTAS group vs. 11.5% MM ($p = 0.009$).
- Any stroke or death within 30 days after enrollment: 14.7% PTAS group vs. 5.8% MM ($p = 0.002$).
- Secondary outcome of any major hemorrhage: 9.8% PTAS group vs. 2.2% MM ($p < 0.001$).

STUDY CONCLUSIONS

Aggressive medical therapy was superior to PTAS (using Wingspan system) in patients with intracranial arterial stenosis. These observations were largely impacted by a high rate of periprocedural stroke after PTAS.

COMMENTARY

The SAMMPRIS trial was performed as the first direct comparison of PTAS to aggressive MM for intracranial arterial stenosis. The significant finding in this study was that maximum medical therapy far outperformed PTAS (with Wingspan system), with a 9% absolute risk reduction for stroke or death. Importantly, the majority of strokes or deaths occurred in the periprocedural period. Of the 33 strokes or deaths that occurred in the PTAS group within 30 days of revascularization, >75% occurred within 1 day after the procedure. After median follow-up of 32.4 months, the early benefit of aggressive medical therapy over stenting with the Wingspan system persisted.[1] One limitation of this study was that MM was only compared to one stenting system, potentially limiting the application to other stent systems. In 2015, however, the VISSIT Trial[2] evaluated balloon-expandable stents (Vitesse Intracranial Stent) in patients with severely stenotic intracranial atherosclerotic lesions, and again MM had lower rates of recurrent stroke or TIA. The results of SAMMPRIS and VISSIT show that percutaneous intervention on intracranial stenosis is harmful. SAMMPRIS revolutionized the approach to management of symptomatic intracranial arterial stenoses with intensive MM.

Question

Is maximum medical therapy for secondary stroke prevention of intracranial atherosclerotic lesions superior to stenting with Wingspan stent system?

Answer

Yes, in patients with symptomatic intracranial stenoses, aggressive medical therapy is superior to stenting.

References

1. Derdeyn CP, Chimowitz MI, Lynn MJ, et al. Aggressive medical treatment with or without stenting in high-risk patients with intracranial artery stenosis (SAMMPRIS): the final results of a randomised trial. *Lancet.* 2014;383(9914):333–341.
2. Zaidat OO, Fitzsimmons B-F, Woodward BK, et al. Effect of a balloon-expandable intracranial stent vs. medical therapy on risk of stroke in patients with symptomatic intracranial stenosis: the VISSIT Randomized Clinical Trial. *JAMA.* 2015;313(12):1240–1248.

| CHAPTER 5 | # WARFARIN FOR ATRIAL FIBRILLATION |

Stroke Prevention in Atrial Fibrillation Study: Final Results

Stroke Prevention in Atrial Fibrillation Investigators. *Circulation*. 1991;84:527–539

BACKGROUND

Atrial fibrillation (AF) increases the risk of ischemic stroke five- to sevenfold because of left atrial thrombus formation and cerebral embolization. Prior to the Stroke Prevention in Atrial Fibrillation (SPAF) study, the efficacy of antithrombotic medications for stroke prevention in patients with AF and absence of cardiac valvular disease had not been firmly established, although smaller trials had suggested a benefit. SPAF was undertaken to evaluate the role of anticoagulant and antiplatelet therapies in a large population of these patients by comparing the outcomes of treatment with warfarin or aspirin compared to placebo.

OBJECTIVES

To evaluate whether treatment with warfarin or aspirin is more effective for preventing ischemic stroke and systemic embolization compared to placebo in patients with nonvalvular AF.

METHODS

Double-blind, placebo-controlled trial conducted at 15 clinical centers between 1987 and 1989.

Patients

1,330 patients with documented AF within 12 months were enrolled if they did not have prosthetic heart valves or evidence of mitral stenosis on echocardiography. A notable exclusion criterion was TIA or ischemic stroke within 2 years.

Interventions

Patients were categorized as either warfarin-eligible or ineligible based on patient preference, hemorrhage risk, and predicted embolization risk. Within the warfarin-eligible group, patients were randomized to warfarin with goal PTT 1.3 to 1.8, aspirin 325 mg daily, or placebo. In the warfarin-ineligible group, patients were randomized to aspirin 325 mg daily or placebo.

Outcomes

The primary outcome was ischemic stroke or systemic embolization over the mean follow-up period of 1.3 years. Secondary outcomes included TIA, MI, death, and unstable angina requiring hospitalization.

KEY RESULTS

- There was a reduction in primary events with aspirin treatment compared to placebo (3.6%/yr vs. 6.3%/yr, RRR = 0.42 [0.09–0.63], p = 0.02). There was also a reduction in rates of primary event or death in the aspirin group (7.9%/yr vs. 11.8%/yr, RRR = 0.32 [0.07–0.50], p = 0.02), but no differences between the groups in other secondary outcomes.
- Warfarin was also associated with decreased primary events compared to placebo (2.3%/yr vs. 7.4%/yr, RRR = 0.67 [0.27–0.85], p = 0.01) and decreased rates of primary events or death (3.8%/yr vs. 9.8%/yr, RRR = 0.58 [0.20–0.78], p = 0.01), but no differences between the groups in other secondary outcomes.
- Rates of major bleeding were similar among the aspirin (1.4%/yr), warfarin (1.5%/yr), and placebo (1.6%/yr) groups.

STUDY CONCLUSIONS

Treatment with aspirin or warfarin is associated with improved outcomes compared to placebo in patients with nonvalvular AF.

COMMENTARY

SPAF was a cardinal study in establishing the benefits of anticoagulation and antiplatelet therapies in reducing embolic complications of nonvalvular AF. Although earlier studies, such as the Danish (AFASAK) and Boston area (BAATAF), had shown a benefit of warfarin use in similar patient populations, SPAF was a much larger trial that also showed a benefit of treatment with aspirin. This study additionally suggested a greater effect with warfarin compared to aspirin (risk reduction of 67% vs. 42%), and these agents were both safe, although the groups were not directly compared. SPAF led to later trials that did compare these agents. The European AF trial showed greater ischemic stroke prevention with warfarin than with aspirin in nonvalvular AF patients. The ACTIVE-W trial showed improved vascular outcomes in nonvalvular AF patients receiving an oral anticoagulant compared to those receiving dual antiplatelet therapy with clopidogrel and aspirin. In the absence of a cardioembolic source such as AF, warfarin has not been found to reduce recurrent stroke rates. For example, the WARSS trial showed no secondary stroke prevention benefit of warfarin over aspirin in patients without AF or another inferred cardioembolic source.

Question

Does treatment with antithrombotic medications decrease ischemic stroke risk in patients with nonvalvular AF?

Answer

Yes, anticoagulation is the most effective treatment for ischemic stroke prevention in these patients, and aspirin has been shown to have a modest benefit.

CHAPTER 6

NOVEL ORAL ANTICOAGULANTS FOR STROKE PREVENTION IN NONVALVULAR ATRIAL FIBRILLATION

Dabigatran versus Warfarin in Patients with Atrial Fibrillation

Connolly SJ, Ezekowitz MD, Yusuf S, et al; RE-LY Steering Committee and Investigators. *NEJM*. 2009;361(12):1139–1151

BACKGROUND

AF is associated with an increased risk of ischemic stroke, and anticoagulant treatment is one of the most effective therapies for reducing this risk. However, vitamin K antagonists increase rates of hemorrhage and can be challenging to maintain within a desired international normalized ratio (INR) range. RE-LY was undertaken to compare an oral anticoagulant agent, the direct thrombin inhibitor dabigatran, with warfarin in patients with nonvalvular AF to determine if this medication had the potential to provide equivalent stroke prevention and decreased bleeding complications.

OBJECTIVES

To compare treatment outcomes with dabigatran and warfarin in patients with nonvalvular AF.

METHODS

Double-blind, randomized trial conducted at 951 clinical centers in 44 countries, with enrollment between 2005 and 2007.

Patients

18,113 patients with AF documented within 6 months were enrolled if they had at least one of the following characteristics: previous TIA or stroke, left ventricular ejection fraction <40%, New York Heart Association class II heart failure symptoms or more severe within 6 months, age > 74 or 65 to 74 years with diabetes, hypertension, or coronary artery disease. Notable exclusion criteria included cardiac valve disease or recent stroke.

Interventions

Patients were randomized to receive dabigatran 110 mg twice daily, dabigatran 150 mg twice daily, or warfarin (titrated to INR 2–3). Concomitant antiplatelet therapy was permitted.

Outcomes

The primary outcome was the composite of stroke or systemic embolism over the median follow-up period of 2 years. The primary safety outcome was major hemorrhage. Secondary outcomes included stroke, systemic embolism, and death.

KEY RESULTS

- Dabigatran 150 mg was superior to warfarin in decreasing primary event rates (1.11%/yr vs. 1.69%/yr, RR = 0.66 [0.53–0.82], $p < 0.001$).

- Dabigatran 110 mg was noninferior to warfarin in primary event rates (1.53%/yr vs. 1.69%/yr, RR = 0.91 [0.74–1.11], $p < 0.001$), but not superior ($p = 0.34$).
- Major bleeding rates were decreased in the dabigatran 110 mg group (2.71%/yr vs. 3.36%/yr, RR = 0.80 [0.69–0.93], $p = 0.003$) but not the 150 mg group (3.11%/yr vs. 3.36%/yr, RR = 0.93 [0.81–1.07], $p = 0.31$) compared to warfarin.
- Intracranial bleeding was reduced in both the dabigatran 150 mg (0.30%/yr vs. 0.74%/yr, RR = 0.40 [0.27–0.60], $p < 0.001$) and 110 mg (0.23%/yr vs. 0.74%/yr, RR = 0.31 [0.20–0.47], $p < 0.001$) groups compared to warfarin.

STUDY CONCLUSIONS

In patients with nonvalvular AF, dabigatran 150 mg was associated with decreased stroke and systemic embolism, decreased intracranial hemorrhage, and equivalent major bleeding rates compared to warfarin. Dabigatran 110 mg was associated with equivalent stroke and systemic embolism rates and decreased rates of intracranial and major bleeding compared to warfarin.

COMMENTARY

RE-LY was the first study to show a benefit of treatment with a novel anticoagulant, in this case dabigatran, when compared with warfarin in patients with nonvalvular AF. The purpose was to determine whether an alternate treatment could provide the same degree of stroke protection but with decreased bleeding rates and avoidance of the need for monitoring blood tests. The positive results led to subsequent trials with similarly improved outcomes when comparing the factor Xa inhibitors to warfarin. Specifically, in ROCKET-AF, rivaroxaban was found to be noninferior to warfarin in stroke and systemic embolism prevention and superior in decreasing rates of intracranial (0.5%/yr vs. 0.7%/yr, $p = 0.02$) and fatal hemorrhages (0.2%/yr vs. 0.5%/yr, $p = 0.003$). ARISTOTLE compared apixaban to warfarin and, in addition to displaying superior stroke, systemic embolism, major bleeding, and intracranial bleeding rates, apixaban showed a mortality benefit over warfarin (3.52% vs. 3.94%, hazard ratio = 0.89 [0.80–0.99], $p = 0.047$). Of note, ARISTOTLE showed superiority of apixaban over warfarin for the end point "all strokes," which included hemorrhagic strokes. This result was due to a reduction in hemorrhagic strokes. Meanwhile, apixaban did not show superiority for ischemic strokes. These trials have led to a major change in the treatment of patients with nonvalvular AF such that clinicians now often prescribe one of the novel anticoagulant medications in favor of warfarin.

Question

Is treatment with a factor II or factor Xa inhibitor a reasonable alternative to warfarin in patients with nonvalvular AF?

Answer

Yes, these medications are associated with similar or improved stroke and systemic embolism rates and decreased bleeding complications compared to warfarin.

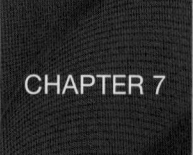

CHAPTER 7

INTENSE LOW-DENSITY LIPOPROTEIN CHOLESTEROL REDUCTION FOR STROKE PREVENTION

High-Dose Atorvastatin after Stroke or Transient Ischemic Attack

SPARCL Investigators. *NEJM*. 2006;355:549–559

BACKGROUND

Prior to SPARCL, there was no compelling evidence to support a role for 3-hydroxy-3-methylglutaryl coenzyme A reductase inhibitors (statins) in secondary prevention of stroke or TIAs among patients previously experiencing a stroke or TIA. The CARE, LIPID, and 4S trials had established a role for statins in the primary prevention of stroke or TIA in patients at high risk of cardiovascular disease. At the time of this study, however, it was uncertain whether statin therapy reduced the risk of recurrent stroke.

OBJECTIVES

To determine whether high-dose statin therapy reduces the risk of stroke in patients with a recent stroke or TIA.

METHODS

Prospective, randomized multicenter trial at 205 centers worldwide from 1998 to 2001.

Patients

4,731 patients with recent (1 to 6 months) ischemic or hemorrhagic stroke or TIA and a cholesterol level between 100 and 190 mg/dL and no known coronary disease were enrolled. Patients were excluded if they had AF or cardiac sources of embolism.

Interventions

Patients were randomly assigned to double-blind therapy with atorvastatin 80 mg/day or placebo.

Outcomes

The primary outcome was the time from randomization to a stroke. Secondary outcomes included TIA, major coronary event (e.g., MI or cardiac arrest), death from cardiac causes, and any revascularization procedure.

KEY RESULTS

- Over 4.9 years, 11.2% in the atorvastatin group vs. 13.1% in the placebo group had a fatal or nonfatal stroke (HR = 0.84, 95% CI = 0.71–0.99, p = 0.03).
- Five-year absolute reduction in risk of major cardiovascular events was 3.5% (HR = 0.80, 95% CI = 0.69–0.92, p = 0.002) in the atorvastatin group.

- Adverse events in the atorvastatin group included increased incidence of alanine transaminase or aspartate aminotransferase greater than three times the upper limit of normal (2.2% vs. 0.5%, $p < 0.001$) and hemorrhagic stroke (HR = 1.66, 95% CI = 1.08–2.55, $p = 0.03$).

STUDY CONCLUSIONS

In patients without known coronary heart disease, treatment with atorvastatin 80 mg daily reduced the risk of subsequent stroke in patients with a recent stroke or TIA and with LDL cholesterol levels between 100 and 190 mg/dL.

COMMENTARY

Prior to SPARCL, no studies had been published showing that statin treatment was beneficial for reducing the risk of recurrent stroke or TIA. Studies like CARE, 4S, and LIPID trials had already established a role for statins in the primary prevention of stroke and TIA among high-risk patients, and these data served as the impetus for the design of SPARCL. The beneficial effects in this study were attributed to dramatically reducing serum LDL cholesterol levels because mean LDL cholesterol levels in the atorvastatin group were 72.9 mg/dL compared to 128.5 mg/dL in the placebo group. This study and others contributed significantly to management practices of aggressive lowering of serum LDL cholesterol levels in patients with a stroke or TIA. An important caveat in this study is that, despite overall risk reduction of recurrent stroke, the atorvastatin group had a significant increase in the incidence of hemorrhagic stroke. Overall, this study supports the principle that aggressive lowering of serum LDL cholesterol in patients with ischemic stroke is beneficial.

Question

Can high-dose statin therapy safely reduce the risk of recurrent stroke or TIA in patients without known coronary heart disease?

Answer

Yes, high-dose statin therapy is efficacious for secondary stroke prevention in patients without known coronary heart disease and LDL cholesterol levels between 100 and 190 mg/dL.

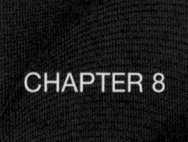

CHAPTER 8

MARGINAL BENEFIT FROM DEVICE CLOSURE OF PATENT FORAMEN OVALE

Closure of Patent Foramen Ovale versus Medical Therapy after Cryptogenic Stroke
Carroll JD, Saver JL, Thaler DE, et al. *NEJM*. 2013;368:1092–1100

BACKGROUND
The optimal management of patent foramen ovale (PFO) in the setting of cryptogenic stroke is unclear. Prior to the publication of RESPECT, it was unclear whether closure of a PFO was efficacious for secondary stroke prevention after a cryptogenic stroke. A randomized trial using the STARFlex septal closure system (CLOSURE I) did not show superiority over medical therapy alone; however, observational studies had shown newer closure devices to have improved safety features.

OBJECTIVES
To evaluate whether closure of a PFO reduces recurrent ischemic stroke when compared to medical therapy.

METHODS
Prospective, multicenter, randomized, open-label trial performed at 69 sites in the United States and Canada between 2003 and 2011.

Patients
980 patients with cryptogenic stroke and PFO demonstrated by transthoracic echocardiogram bubble study were randomized. Notably, patients were excluded from the trial if a mechanism other than paradoxical embolism could be identified for the index stroke.

Interventions
Medical therapy group consisted of aspirin, clopidogrel, warfarin, or combination of aspirin and extended-release dipyridamole. Patients in closure group underwent Amplatzer PFO Occluder insertion followed by aspirin plus clopidogrel for 1 month and subsequently aspirin monotherapy for 5 months.

Outcomes
Primary end point was a composite of recurrent fatal ischemic stroke, nonfatal ischemic stroke, or death within 30 to 45 days after randomization. Secondary end points included complete closure of PFO on 6-month follow-up, absence of a TIA, or recurrent symptomatic nonfatal ischemic stroke or cardiovascular death.

KEY RESULTS
- In the intention-to-treat group, 25 primary end-point events occurred (all nonfatal ischemic strokes); 9 closure group vs. 16 medical therapy group (HR = 0.49, 95% CI = 0.22–1.11, p = 0.08).

- In the as-treated analysis, PFO closure was superior to medical therapy (6 vs. 14 events, HR = 0.37, 95% CI = 0.14–0.96, p = 0.03).
- There was no difference in rates of secondary outcomes (TIA or composite recurrent symptomatic nonfatal ischemic stroke or cardiovascular mortality) between the groups.
- Subgroup analysis demonstrated that management of substantial shunts (0.8% vs 4.3%, HR = 0.18, 95% CI = 0.04–0.81, p = 0.01) and atrial septal aneurysms (1.1% vs. 5.3%, HR = 0.19, 95% CI = 0.04–0.87, p = 0.02) favored closure.

STUDY CONCLUSIONS

In the primary intention-to-treat cohort, there was no significant benefit from closure of a PFO in adults with cryptogenic stroke.

COMMENTARY

The RESPECT study was undertaken to assess whether improved PFO closure devices reduced recurrent stroke in patients with cryptogenic stroke compared to medical therapy alone. Prior to RESPECT, CLOSURE I had shown that PFO closure with the STARFlex closure device was not superior to medical therapy alone for recurrent stroke prevention and was associated with higher rates of AF and atrial thrombus. The question of the potential benefit of PFO closure was not fully settled by RESPECT. The PC Trial, which used the same closure device as RESPECT, affirmed the findings of RESPECT that despite high rates of PFO closure, intervention was not strictly superior to medical therapy alone in an intention-to-treat analysis. Yet, the positive findings of RESPECT kept the question of potential benefit in some subgroups alive. These findings warrant further consideration: (1) that PFO closure was superior to medical therapy in the per-protocol and as-treated analyses, (2) that on subgroup analysis, PFO closure was superior when atrial septal aneurysms or large shunts were present. The criticisms of RESPECT are related to its uneven dropout rates between groups and unblinded event adjudication. Ultimately, the decision to close PFOs in patients with cryptogenic stroke remains uncertain, with clinical decision making performed on an individual patient basis dependent on patient and PFO characteristics.

Question

Does PFO closure reduce the risk of recurrent stroke in patients with cryptogenic stroke compared to medical therapy alone?

Answer

No, the RESPECT and PC Trial showed that in the intention-to-treat cohort, PFO closure was not superior to medical therapy for secondary stroke prevention.

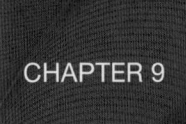

CHAPTER 9

EARLY DECOMPRESSIVE SURGERY IN MALIGNANT INFARCTION OF THE MIDDLE CEREBRAL ARTERY

Early Decompressive Surgery in Malignant Infarction of the Middle Cerebral Artery: A Pooled Analysis of Three Randomized Controlled Trials

Vahedi K, Hofmeijer J, Juettler E, et al. *Lancet Neurol*. 2007;6:215–222

BACKGROUND

The abysmal prognosis of and absence of any efficacious medical treatment for malignant middle cerebral artery (MCA) ischemic strokes prompted investigators to explore the benefit with surgical decompression. Prior to DECIMAL, DESTINY, and HAMLET, several nonrandomized studies suggested that decompressive hemicraniectomy reduced mortality. DECIMAL, DESTINY, and HAMLET were the first three randomized trials to evaluate a role for decompressive surgery in the management of malignant MCA infarctions.

OBJECTIVES

To perform a pooled analysis of three RCTs on decompressive surgery in malignant MCA infarction, and to assess whether surgical intervention improved functional outcomes and mortality.

METHODS

Three multicenter, randomized controlled clinical trials conducted in Germany, France, and the Netherlands with enrollment between 2001 and 2006 (DESTINY 2004–2005, HAMLET 2002–2006, DECIMAL 2001–2005).

Patients

Ninety-three patients aged 18 to 60 years with MCA infarct exceeding 50% of the territory, NIHSS > 15, inclusion within 45 hours of symptom onset, and decreased consciousness as assessed by score of 1 or greater on item 1a of NIHSS were included in the pooled analysis. Notable exclusion criteria included life expectancy less than 3 years, baseline mRS ≥ 2, and hemorrhagic transformation of the infarct.

Interventions

Patients in the decompressive surgery group were treated with a large bone flap and duroplasty. No brain tissue was resected. Patients in the conservative treatment group received standard stroke care and antiedema treatment.

Outcomes

The primary outcome measure was mRS score at 1 year dichotomized as favorable (mRS 0 to 4) or unfavorable (mRS 5 and 6). Secondary outcomes included a second dichotomization of mRS at 1 year into 0 to 3 and >4 and 1 year mortality.

KEY RESULTS
- Patients in the decompressive surgery group were more likely to achieve a favorable outcome than those in the conservative treatment group (mRS > 4: 13/51 (25%) vs. 32/42 (76%) patients, 95% CI = 33.9–68.5, OR = 0.10).
- The surgery group had significantly higher rates of mRS 2 to 3 at 12 months: 22/51 (43%) vs. 9/42 (21%) patients (95% CI = 4.6–40.9, OR = 0.13–0.86).
- There were significantly fewer deaths at 12 months in the surgery group: 11/51 (22%) vs. 30/42 (71%) patients (95% CI = 0.04–0.27, OR = 0.10).

STUDY CONCLUSIONS
In patients with malignant MCA infarction that are less than 60 years old, decompressive surgery performed within 48 hours of stroke onset reduces mortality and increases the likelihood of a favorable outcome.

COMMENTARY

The trials DECIMAL, DESTINY, and HAMLET were pursued to evaluate the role of decompressive surgery to improve outcomes and reduce mortality in patients with malignant MCA infarctions. The pooled results of these studies were dramatic, showing that with the appropriate selection criteria, only 2.4 people needed to undergo surgery to save one life. DESTINY II expanded this investigation to evaluate patients aged 61 years or older. In patients >61 years of age, decompressive surgery reduces mortality (33% vs. 70%), but, unlike the findings of DESTINY, DECIMAL, and HAMLET, it does not increase the rate of favorable functional outcomes. (No patient attained mRS score of 0 to 2 at 12 months in DESTINY II.) Thus, although these studies demonstrated a pronounced effect on patients less than 60 years old with stroke, it is critical to evaluate patient candidacy for decompressive surgery on an individual basis. These studies revolutionized the treatment of malignant MCA infarction by showing that the appropriately selected patient will strongly benefit from surgery.

Question
Does hemicraniectomy for malignant MCA infarction improve the likelihood of favorable functional outcomes and reduce mortality?

Answer
Yes, in patients less than 60 years of age, urgent decompressive surgery improves functional outcomes and reduces mortality at 12 months.

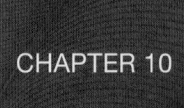

CHAPTER 10
CAROTID ENDARTERECTOMY FOR STROKE PREVENTION IN INTERNAL CAROTID ARTERY STENOSIS

Beneficial Effect of Carotid Endarterectomy in Symptomatic Patients with High-Grade Carotid Stenosis

North American Symptomatic Carotid Endarterectomy Trial Collaborators. *NEJM.* 1991;325(7):445–453

BACKGROUND

Carotid endarterectomy for stroke prevention in internal carotid artery stenosis had been performed for over three decades prior to the NASCET study. However, trials evaluating its efficacy had shown mixed results, and with the increasing use of antiplatelet therapy for secondary stroke prevention, it was unclear which patients, if any, would benefit from this procedure. To determine its utility, the NASCET trial evaluated the use of carotid endarterectomy compared to MM in a targeted population that would be most likely to benefit, those with >70% internal carotid stenosis and recent ipsilateral ischemic stroke or TIA.

OBJECTIVES

To evaluate whether carotid endarterectomy is more effective than MM alone for ischemic stroke prevention in patients with high-grade symptomatic internal carotid artery stenosis.

METHODS

Randomized trial conducted at 50 medical centers in the United States and Canada between 1988 and 1991 (randomization was stopped early because of evidence of surgical treatment efficacy in patients with high-grade stenosis).

Patients

659 patients with 70% to 99% internal carotid artery stenosis by angiogram were enrolled if they had an ipsilateral hemispheric or retinal TIA or ipsilateral nondisabling ischemic stroke within 120 days. Notable exclusion criteria included carotid disease or symptoms not attributable to atherosclerosis or comorbid cardiac valve or rhythm disorders increasing the risk of cardioembolism.

Interventions

All patients received aspirin 1,300 mg daily unless a lower dose was necessary because of side effects, as well as treatment for hypertension, hyperlipidemia, and/or diabetes as indicated. Patients were randomized to this treatment alone or in conjunction with carotid endarterectomy. Surgery was performed at experienced centers with specified low rates of complications.

Outcomes

The primary outcome was any fatal or nonfatal stroke ipsilateral to the carotid stenosis over a mean follow-up period of 18 months. Secondary outcomes included all strokes, all deaths, and stroke severity (major strokes were defined as those that caused functional deficits lasting >90 days).

KEY RESULTS

- Ipsilateral stroke rates: 9.0% in surgical vs. 26.0% in medical group (ARR = 17 ± 3.5% [SE], $p < 0.001$).
- Major or fatal ipsilateral stroke rates: 2.5% in surgical vs. 13.1% in medical group (ARR = 10.6 ± 2.6% [SE], $p < 0.001$).
- The surgical group had significantly lower rates of any stroke, any stroke or death, any major or fatal stroke, and any major stroke or death compared to the medical group ($p < 0.01$).

STUDY CONCLUSIONS

In patients with recently symptomatic and high-grade (>70%) internal carotid artery stenosis, carotid endarterectomy reduces stroke and mortality rates compared to medical therapy alone.

COMMENTARY

The NASCET trial was pursued to determine the role of carotid endarterectomy in the treatment of patients with symptomatic high-grade internal carotid artery stenosis. The study showed a clear benefit of surgery in these patients in preventing strokes, disabling strokes, and mortality, and the perioperative risk associated with the procedure was overcome by a sustained benefit only 3 months after randomization. NASCET II then showed that patients with symptomatic moderate carotid stenosis of 50% to 69% also had decreased recurrent stroke rates with surgery, although to a lesser degree (5-year ipsilateral stroke rate of 15.7% vs. 22.2% in the medical group, $p = 0.045$, NNT 15). Patients with symptomatic carotid stenosis <50% did not have improved outcomes with surgery. Taken together, these trials were pivotal for guiding clinical practice by establishing carotid endarterectomy as an effective treatment for stroke prevention in patients with symptomatic carotid stenosis and showing that the benefit associated with the procedure was likely based on the degree of stenosis.

Question

Does carotid endarterectomy reduce the risk of stroke in patients with symptomatic high-grade internal carotid artery stenosis?

Answer

Yes, patients with symptomatic carotid stenosis >70% have a dramatic decrease in stroke risk following carotid endarterectomy, and patients with symptomatic carotid stenosis 50% to 69% derive a more modest benefit.

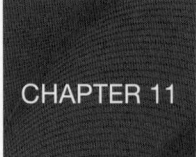

CHAPTER 11

CAROTID ARTERY STENTING VS. CAROTID ENDARTERECTOMY FOR SYMPTOMATIC AND ASYMPTOMATIC CAROTID ARTERY STENOSIS

Stenting versus Endarterectomy for Treatment of Carotid-artery Stenosis

Brott TG, Hobson RW II, Howard G, et al; CREST Investigators. *NEJM.*
2010;363(1):11–23

BACKGROUND

Carotid endarterectomy (CEA) had been shown to be beneficial for stroke prevention both in symptomatic and asymptomatic high-grade internal carotid artery stenosis. However, prior to the CREST trial, it was unclear how carotid stenting compared to CEA in these patients because small trials had shown conflicting results. CREST was a large-scale trial undertaken to determine if carotid artery stenting (CAS) was in fact a safe and effective alternative to CEA.

OBJECTIVES

To compare the outcomes of CAS with those of CEA among patients with symptomatic or asymptomatic high-grade carotid stenosis.

METHODS

Prospective, randomized trial conducted at 117 medical centers in the United States and Canada between December 2000 and July 2008.

Patients

2,502 patients with symptomatic (within 180 days) or asymptomatic internal carotid artery stenosis were enrolled if symptomatic carotid stenosis was >50% on angiography or >70% on carotid ultrasound, CTA, or MRA and asymptomatic carotid stenosis was >60% on angiography, >70% on ultrasound, or >80% on CTA or MRA. Notable exclusion criteria included previous disabling stroke, AF, or recent cardiac ischemia.

Interventions

Patients were randomized to undergo CEA or CAS with the RX Acculink stent. The procedure was performed within 2 weeks of randomization. Patients in the CEA group received aspirin 325 mg daily prior to the procedure and extending for at least 1 year. Those in the CAS group received aspirin 325 mg and clopidogrel 75 mg twice daily before the procedure and daily or twice daily for at least 1 month after the procedure. Other antiplatelet regimens were alternatives.

Outcomes

The primary outcome was the composite of any ischemic stroke, MI, or death during the periprocedural period (30 days after procedure) or ipsilateral ischemic stroke within a 4-year follow-up period (median 2.5 years). Secondary outcomes included components of the primary outcome as well as minor, major, or any stroke.

KEY RESULTS

- There was no difference between CAS and CEA in estimated 4-year rates of the primary outcome (7.2% vs. 6.8%, HR = 1.11 [0.81–1.51], p = 0.51) or during the periprocedural period (5.2% vs. 4.5%, HR = 1.18 [0.82–1.68], p = 0.38).
- Rates of periprocedural stroke were higher in the CAS than in the CEA group (4.1% vs. 2.3%, HR = 1.79 [1.14–2.82], p = 0.01).
- Rates of periprocedural MI were lower in the CAS than in the CEA group (1.1% vs. 2.3%, HR = 0.50 [0.26–0.94], p = 0.03).
- After the periprocedural period, ipsilateral stroke rates were similar in the CAS and CEA groups (2.0% vs. 2.4%, p = 0.85).

STUDY CONCLUSIONS

In patients with high-grade symptomatic or asymptomatic carotid stenosis, overall outcomes between CEA and CAS were similar.

COMMENTARY

The CREST trial was performed to compare the safety and efficacy of carotid stenting with CEA in patients with high-grade carotid stenosis. Results showed that the two interventions had counterbalancing benefits. That is, carotid stenting resulted in fewer periprocedural myocardial infarctions, whereas CEA resulted in fewer periprocedural strokes, leading to similar 4-year rates of the primary outcome. There were also no differences in outcome between the groups in patients with symptomatic or asymptomatic carotid disease. These findings were important, establishing carotid stenting as a viable alternative to CEA and making it an attractive option for patients with high surgical risk.

Question

Are the outcome benefits between CEA and carotid stenting similar in patients with high-grade internal carotid artery stenosis?

Answer

Yes, outcomes were similar between the procedures, with decreased rates of periprocedural stroke associated with CEA balancing the decreased rates of periprocedural MI associated with CAS.

CHAPTER 12

WARFARIN AND ASPIRIN IN PATIENTS WITH HEART FAILURE AND SINUS RHYTHM

Warfarin and Aspirin in Patients with Heart Failure and Sinus Rhythm

Homma S, Thompson JL, Pullicino PM, et al; WARCEF Investigators. *NEJM.* 2012;366(20):1859–1869

BACKGROUND

Systolic heart failure is a known risk factor for left ventricular thrombus formation and cerebral embolism. Prior to the WARCEF trial, smaller studies had shown a reduction in embolic events and death with anticoagulant use in these patients, but several of the patients in these trials also had AF or valvular heart disease. Other studies compared the use of anticoagulants to aspirin in heart failure patients, but were too small to show conclusive superiority of either agent. The WARCEF trial was a larger scale study designed to evaluate whether warfarin or aspirin was the optimal antithrombotic choice in patients with nonvalvular systolic heart failure and no cardiac arrhythmias.

OBJECTIVES

To determine whether warfarin or aspirin is the preferred treatment for patients in sinus rhythm with reduced left ventricular ejection fraction (LVEF).

METHODS

Double-blind, double-dummy design trial conducted at 168 centers in 11 countries with patient recruitment between 2002 and 2010.

Patients

2,305 patients with LVEF < 36% or wall motion index <1.3 assessed within 3 months were enrolled if they were also in normal sinus rhythm. Patients were excluded if they had valvular cardiac disease or a clear indication for either warfarin or aspirin.

Interventions

Patients were randomized to either warfarin (target INR 2 to 3.5) or aspirin 325 mg daily. Patients were also given a placebo pill of the other treatment, and those in the aspirin group were given fabricated INR results during the study.

Outcomes

The primary outcome was the composite of ischemic stroke, intracerebral hemorrhage, or death from any cause over a mean follow-up period of 3.5 years. The main secondary outcome was a composite of the primary outcome, MI, or hospitalization for heart failure.

KEY RESULTS

- There was no difference in primary outcome rates between the groups (7.47 events per 100 patient-years with warfarin vs. 7.93 with aspirin, HR = 0.93, 95% CI = 0.79–1.10, p = 0.40).
- Rates of ischemic stroke were reduced with warfarin (0.72 events per 100 patient-years vs. 1.36 with aspirin, HR = 0.52, 95% CI = 0.33–0.82, p = 0.005).
- Overall rates of major hemorrhage were higher with warfarin (1.78 events per 100 patient-years vs. 0.87 with aspirin, ARR = 2.05, 95% CI = 1.36–3.12, $p <$ 0.001).
- There were no differences in intracerebral hemorrhage between the groups (0.27 events per 100 patient-years with warfarin vs. 0.22 with aspirin, p = 0.82).
- In a time-varying analysis, warfarin showed a small benefit with time, and HR favored warfarin by the fourth year of follow-up (HR = 0.76, p = 0.04).

STUDY CONCLUSIONS

In patients with normal sinus rhythm and systolic heart failure, warfarin reduces ischemic stroke rates compared to aspirin, but is associated with an increased risk of major hemorrhage.

COMMENTARY

The WARCEF trial evaluated the role of warfarin in patients with systolic heart failure but no other major risk factors for cardioembolism. Similar to the earlier WATCH trial, it was considered to be an equivocal study, because the benefit in ischemic stroke prevention with warfarin compared to aspirin was largely offset by its increased hemorrhage risk. However, there was a slight time-dependent benefit of warfarin use, and the hemorrhage risk was not driven by intracerebral bleeding but rather by systemic bleeding, such as gastrointestinal hemorrhage. Given these findings, a later subgroup analysis of WARCEF was performed and showed that patients under the age of 60 years experienced a significant benefit in primary outcome rates with warfarin compared to aspirin (4.81 vs. 6.76 events per 100 patient-years: HR = 0.63; 95% CI = 0.48–0.84; p = 0.001). These findings were likely attributable to a decrease in all-cause mortality from lower bleeding rates, given that there was no difference in the incidence of major hemorrhage among the younger patients taking warfarin or aspirin. Taken together, these findings showed that warfarin is superior to aspirin for ischemic stroke prevention in patients with systolic heart failure. The increased hemorrhage risk offsets this benefit in patients as a whole, but younger patients may derive an overall benefit, because they are generally less prone to bleeding at baseline.

Question

Can aspirin be used instead of warfarin in the prevention of ischemic stroke among patients over 60 years with normal sinus rhythm and systolic heart failure?

Answer

Yes, although there is no strong evidence in favor of one agent over the other given that the lower ischemic stroke rates associated with warfarin use are offset by increased hemorrhagic complications.

| CHAPTER 13 | SHORT-TERM DUAL ANTIPLATELET THERAPY FOR STROKE PREVENTION AFTER TIA OR MINOR STROKE |

Clopidogrel with Aspirin in Acute Minor Stroke or Transient Ischemic Attack

Wang Y, Wang Y, Zhao X, et al; CHANCE Investigators. *NEJM*. 2013;369(1):11–19

BACKGROUND

The risk of recurrent stroke following TIA or minor ischemic stroke is high, with 10% to 20% of patients having another event within 3 months. Aspirin was shown to have a modest benefit in secondary stroke prevention in these patients. Long-term dual antiplatelet therapy was not shown to add benefit when compared with single antiplatelet therapy. Prior to the CHANCE trial, however, studies had not evaluated whether short-term dual antiplatelet therapy started in the acute setting would have a benefit over single-agent use.

OBJECTIVES

To determine whether a 3-week course of dual antiplatelet therapy started within 24 hours of TIA or minor ischemic stroke was superior to aspirin alone in secondary stroke prevention.

METHODS

Double-blind, placebo-controlled trial conducted at 114 medical centers in China between 2009 and 2012.

Patients

5,170 patients with minor stroke (defined as NIHSS < 4) or moderate- to high-risk TIA (defined as $ABCD^2$ score > 3) were enrolled if symptom onset was within 24 hours. Patients were excluded if they had isolated sensory, visual, or vertiginous symptoms without infarction on head CT or magnetic resonance imaging (MRI), mRS > 2, history of intracranial hemorrhage, or recent gastrointestinal hemorrhage or anticoagulant use.

Interventions

Both groups received aspirin (75 to 300 mg) on day 1. Patients in the clopidogrel–aspirin group received a loading dose of 300 mg of clopidogrel followed by 75 mg daily for 90 days plus aspirin 75 mg daily to complete 21 days. Patients in the aspirin-only group received aspirin 75 mg daily to complete 90 days.

Outcomes

The primary outcome was stroke (ischemic or hemorrhagic) over the 90-day trial period. Secondary outcomes included a new vascular event (ischemic stroke, hemorrhagic stroke, MI, or death caused by stroke), systemic hemorrhage, congestive heart failure, pulmonary embolism, sudden death, or arrhythmia.

KEY RESULTS

- Total stroke rates: 8.2% clopidogrel–aspirin vs. 11.7% aspirin (HR = 0.68, 95% CI = 0.57–0.81, $p < 0.001$).
- Ischemic stroke rates: 7.9% clopidogrel–aspirin vs. 11.4% aspirin (HR = 0.67, 95% CI = 0.56–0.81, $p < 0.001$).
- Hemorrhagic stroke rates: 0.3% clopidogrel–aspirin vs. 0.3% aspirin (HR = 1.01, 95% CI = 0.38–2.70, $p = 0.98$).
- Fatal or disabling stroke rates: 5.2% clopidogrel–aspirin vs. 6.8% aspirin (HR = 0.75, 95% CI = 0.60–0.94, $p = 0.01$).
- Composite of vascular events: 8.4% clopidogrel–aspirin vs. 11.9% aspirin (HR = 0.69, 95% CI = 0.58–0.82, $p < 0.001$).
- There were no significant differences between the groups in severe, moderate, or mild bleeding.

STUDY CONCLUSIONS

In patients with minor ischemic stroke or TIA, treating acutely with a short course of dual antiplatelet therapy is associated with decreased recurrent stroke rates and equivalent bleeding risk compared with aspirin alone.

COMMENTARY

The CHANCE trial was conducted to evaluate whether a short course of dual antiplatelet therapy started immediately following TIA or minor ischemic stroke could improve secondary prevention compared with aspirin alone. The results did show a benefit with dual antiplatelet therapy, and in contrast to MATCH and PRoFESS, which included longer treatment periods, there was no associated increased bleeding risk in the dual antiplatelet group in CHANCE. In addition, a follow-up analysis showed that the early benefit of short-term dual antiplatelet therapy in reducing the risk of subsequent stroke persisted at 1-year follow-up (10.6% vs. 14%).[1] The benefit seen in CHANCE was likely owing to the immediacy of treatment initiation, because the curves for stroke-free survival between the groups separated dramatically in the first few days, after which rates were similar. The study population's demographics were another potential contributor to the observed beneficial effect. For example, there are high rates of stroke and intracranial atherosclerosis in China. Secondary prevention measures, such as treatment of hypertension, diabetes, and hyperlipidemia, are also less frequent. Thus, the results of this study may not be generalizable to other patient populations. The POINT trial, a large multinational study being undertaken to examine the potential benefits of short-term dual antiplatelet treatment in the acute setting, aims to address this question.

Question

Does a short course of dual antiplatelet therapy with clopidogrel and aspirin started within 24 hours of TIA or minor ischemic stroke prevent recurrent strokes to a greater degree than aspirin alone?

Answer

Yes, a 3-week course of clopidogrel and aspirin was associated with decreased stroke rates and similar bleeding risk at 90 days compared to aspirin.

Reference

1. Wang Y, Pan Y, Zhao Z, et al. Clopidogrel with aspirin in acute minor stroke or transient ischemic attack (CHANCE) trial: one-year outcomes. *Circulation*. 2015;132:40–46.

CHAPTER 14

ASPIRIN OVER WARFARIN FOR SYMPTOMATIC INTRACRANIAL STENOSIS

Comparison of Warfarin and Aspirin for Symptomatic Intracranial Arterial Stenosis

Chimowitz MI, Lynn MJ, Howlett-Smith H, et al; Warfarin-Aspirin Symptomatic Intracranial Disease Trial Investigators. *NEJM.* 2005;352(13):1305–1316

BACKGROUND

Atherosclerotic intracranial arterial stenosis is a frequent cause of ischemic stroke, accounting for up to 10% of cases and with a high recurrence rate. However, prior to the WASID study, there were no prospective trials comparing the efficacy of different antithrombotic agents for the treatment of these patients. To answer the question of whether anticoagulation or antiplatelet therapy is the optimal treatment strategy, WASID compared treatment with warfarin versus aspirin in patients with recent TIA or ischemic stroke in the setting of >50% stenosis of a major intracranial artery.

OBJECTIVES

To compare outcomes of treatment with warfarin versus aspirin for patients with symptomatic intracranial arterial stenosis.

METHODS

Double-blind, placebo-controlled trial conducted at 59 clinical sites in North America between 1999 and 2003 (enrollment stopped early because of safety concerns with warfarin treatment).

Patients

569 patients with TIA or nondisabling ischemic stroke within 90 days were enrolled if they had angiogram-confirmed 50% to 99% stenosis of the carotid, middle cerebral, vertebral, or basilar artery. Notable exclusion criteria included a modified Rankin score >3, cardioembolic source (such as AF), or tandem >50% stenoses of the extracranial carotid artery.

Interventions

Patients were randomized to receive either warfarin (titrated to INR 2 to 3) or aspirin 650 mg twice daily during the study period. Aspirin could be lowered to 325 mg twice daily if patients experienced side effects. Both groups received placebo pills representing the other treatment and underwent monthly INR checks.

Outcomes

The primary outcome was the composite of ischemic stroke, intracerebral hemorrhage, and death from vascular causes other than stroke over the mean follow-up period of 1.8 years. Secondary outcomes included components of the primary outcome, as well as ischemic stroke in the territory of the stenotic artery, and disabling or fatal ischemic stroke.

KEY RESULTS

- There was no difference between the aspirin and warfarin groups in the rates of primary outcome (22.1% vs. 21.8%, HR = 1.04 [0.73–1.48], p = 0.83).
- There were no significant differences between the groups on any of the secondary outcomes.
- Aspirin was associated with decreased rates of multiple adverse events compared to warfarin, including major hemorrhage (3.2% vs. 8.3%, HR = 0.39 [0.18–0.84], p = 0.01), MI or sudden death (2.9% vs. 7.3%, HR = 0.40 [0.18–0.91], p = 0.02), and death from any cause (4.3% vs. 9.7%, HR = 0.46 [0.23–0.90], p = 0.02), although not death from vascular causes (3.2% vs. 5.9%, HR = 0.56 [0.25–1.26], p = 0.16).

STUDY CONCLUSIONS

In patients with recent TIA or ischemic stroke and significant major intracranial artery stenosis, treatment with warfarin is no better than with aspirin and is associated with higher rates of adverse events.

COMMENTARY

The WASID trial was conducted to evaluate whether anticoagulation or antiplatelet therapy was the more appropriate treatment for symptomatic major intracranial artery stenosis. The study was stopped early, because warfarin was shown not to improve outcomes compared to aspirin and to be associated with high rates of multiple adverse events, including death. These results have had a significant impact on clinical practice, because prior to this study, experts were divided on whether to treat these patients with anticoagulation or antiplatelet therapy. However, WASID did not settle the question in all cases. The adverse events related to warfarin use were a result of systemic rather than neurovascular outcomes, which may confer a high rate of disability, and a lenient definition of major hemorrhage may have worsened the warfarin results. There were no differences between the groups in intracranial hemorrhage, ischemic stroke, or death from vascular causes. Yet a critique accompanying the study noted that patients who achieved a therapeutic INR had much lower rates of ischemic stroke.[1] A later subgroup analysis showed that there may be a role for warfarin use in certain populations of patients with major intracranial artery stenosis given that primary outcomes were superior with warfarin treatment compared to aspirin in patients with symptomatic basilar artery stenosis (HR = 2.28 [1.02–5.08], p = 0.044), although warfarin conferred no benefit for ischemic stroke in the territory of the symptomatic basilar artery. There was also a trend toward higher primary event rates in those randomized to aspirin <18 days after the index event (HR = 1.55 [0.98–2.44], p = 0.06).

Question

Should treatment with aspirin be used over warfarin in patients with recent TIA or ischemic stroke and major intracranial arterial stenosis?

Answer

Yes, aspirin is the preferred treatment in most cases, because it has similar efficacy and fewer adverse events compared to warfarin's use in common practice. Yet there may be a benefit of warfarin in patients with basilar artery stenosis, and treatment decisions in all patients should be individualized.

Reference

1. Koroshetz WJ. Warfarin, aspirin, and intracranial vascular disease. *NEJM*. 2005;352:1368–1370.

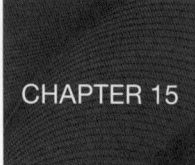

LACK OF BENEFIT FROM LONG-TERM DUAL ANTIPLATELET THERAPY FOR SECONDARY STROKE PREVENTION

Aspirin and Clopidogrel Compared with Clopidogrel Alone after Recent Ischaemic Stroke or Transient Ischaemic Attack in High-Risk Patients (MATCH): Randomized, Double-Blind, Placebo-Controlled Trial

Diener HC, Bogousslavsky J, Brass LM, et al; MATCH Investigators. *Lancet.* 2004;364(9431):331–337

BACKGROUND

Antiplatelet therapy with a single agent has been shown to be beneficial for secondary prevention in patients with ischemic stroke or TIA. Studies have also shown that in patients with coronary atherothrombotic disease, addition of clopidogrel to aspirin results in improved outcomes compared to single antiplatelet therapy. The MATCH trial was designed to answer the question of whether dual antiplatelet therapy with clopidogrel and aspirin could show a similar benefit in reducing recurrent ischemic events in patients following ischemic stroke or TIA compared to treatment with clopidogrel alone.

OBJECTIVES

To evaluate whether dual antiplatelet therapy improves outcomes compared to clopidogrel following ischemic stroke or TIA.

METHODS

Double-blind, placebo-controlled trial conducted at 507 medical centers in 28 countries between 2000 and 2003.

Patients

7,599 patients with acute ischemic stroke or TIA within 3 months were enrolled if they had at least one other vascular risk factor. Notable exclusion criteria were severe comorbid conditions and those that increased bleeding risk.

Interventions

Patients were randomized to aspirin 75 mg daily or placebo for 18 months. All patients also received clopidogrel 75 mg daily during the trial period.

Outcomes

The primary outcome was the composite of ischemic stroke, MI, vascular death, or rehospitalization for an acute ischemic event (including TIA, unstable angina, or worsening peripheral vascular disease requiring therapeutic intervention). Secondary outcomes included components of the primary outcome, death from any cause, and any stroke.

KEY RESULTS

- There was no significant difference between primary outcome events in the clopidogrel–aspirin vs. clopidogrel groups (15.7% vs. 16.7% patients, $p = 0.244$).
- There were no differences between the groups in any of the secondary outcomes.
- There was an increased major bleeding risk in the clopidogrel–aspirin group compared to the clopidogrel group (1.9% vs. 0.6%, $p < 0.0001$).
- Life-threatening bleeding rates were also higher in the clopidogrel–aspirin group compared to the clopidogrel group (2.6% vs. 1.3%, $p < 0.0001$).

STUDY CONCLUSIONS

Continuous dual antiplatelet therapy with clopidogrel and aspirin is no better than clopidogrel alone for the prevention of ischemic events in patients with recent ischemic stroke or TIA and is associated with a higher bleeding risk.

COMMENTARY

The MATCH trial was performed to evaluate whether long-term dual antiplatelet therapy was more effective than single-agent treatment for secondary prevention in patients with recent ischemic stroke or TIA. The results showed not only a lack of added benefit of dual antiplatelet treatment in preventing ischemic events, but also an associated increased risk of significant bleeding compared to single-agent use. Subsequent studies showed similar findings. For example, CHARISMA showed a lack of benefit with clopidogrel and aspirin use compared to aspirin alone in a population at high risk for atherothrombotic disease, and PRoFESS showed no added benefit in secondary stroke prevention with aspirin and dipyridamole compared to clopidogrel in addition to greater risk of major hemorrhage and intracranial hemorrhage in the dual antiplatelet group. The findings from these studies were important in guiding clinical practice, because they showed lack of efficacy and potential for harm from use of long-term dual antiplatelet therapy for secondary stroke prevention.

Question

Does prolonged dual antiplatelet therapy improve outcomes compared to single-agent use in patients with ischemic stroke or TIA?

Answer

No, long-term dual antiplatelet therapy is no more effective and increases the risk of major hemorrhage compared to treatment with a single antiplatelet agent.

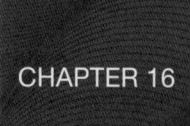
FLUOXETINE FOR MOTOR RECOVERY AFTER ACUTE ISCHEMIC STROKE

Fluoxetine for Motor Recovery after Acute Ischaemic Stroke (FLAME): A Randomised Placebo-Controlled Trial

Chollet F, Tardy J, Albucher J-F, et al. *Lancet Neurol.* 2011;10:123–130

BACKGROUND

Acute ischemic stroke represents a major cause of long-term disability, with two-thirds of stroke survivors having residual neurologic impairment and more than a quarter dependent in activities of daily living. Prior to the FLAME trial, several small case series had suggested a beneficial role for early administration of selective serotonin reuptake inhibitors to modulate motor recovery. FLAME was a large-scale trial to evaluate the safety of fluoxetine and assess its role in enhancing motor recovery.

OBJECTIVES

To evaluate whether a 3-month treatment with fluoxetine would enhance motor recovery for patients with acute ischemic stroke and moderate to severe motor deficits.

METHODS

Double-blind, placebo-controlled trial conducted at nine stroke centers in France between 2005 and 2009.

Patients

118 patients with an acute ischemic stroke within the past 5 to 10 days and resultant hemiparesis were enrolled if baseline Fugl–Meyer motor scale (FMMS) scores were 55 or less. Patients were excluded if there was significant premorbid disability, NIHSS >20, depression, or other preexisting deficits that could interfere with assessments.

Interventions

Patients were randomized to 20 mg fluoxetine daily or placebo for 90 days. All patients received physiotherapy during the treatment period. The analysis was adjusted for patient age, history of stroke, and baseline mRS or NIHSS scores.

Outcomes

Primary outcome was the mean change in FMMS score over 90 days. Secondary end points included change in NIHSS, modified Rankin scale, and Montgomery–Åsberg depression rating scale over the 90-day period.

KEY RESULTS

- The adjusted mean change in FMMS score was significantly higher in the fluoxetine group than in the placebo group (34.0 vs. 24.3, 95% CI = 3.4–16.1, p = 0.003).
- There was no difference in total NIHSS score at 90 days between the groups; however, motor scores were significantly reduced in the fluoxetine group (4.7 vs. 6.3, p = 0.012).
- There was a significant increase in number of patients scored as independent on mRS (e.g., 0 to 2) in the fluoxetine group (adjusted mean 34% vs. 11%, p = 0.021).
- The rate of depression was higher in the placebo group than in the fluoxetine group (29% vs. 7%, p = 0.002).

STUDY CONCLUSIONS

In patients with acute ischemic stroke, a positive effect on motor recovery, as assessed by change in FMMS score, was observed with fluoxetine treatment for 90 days.

COMMENTARY

The FLAME trial was undertaken to evaluate whether fluoxetine therapy in combination with intensive poststroke rehabilitation could augment motor recovery. The trial succeeded in showing that fluoxetine treatment is safe, potentially improves motor recovery, and also reduces the incidence of poststroke depression. This trial has had a great impact on clinical practice: the initiation of fluoxetine in the poststroke period is now commonplace. The mechanism underlying the clinical effect remains unclear. The effect of fluoxetine may be mediated through brain-derived neurotrophic factor upregulation and synaptic rewiring, as has been demonstrated at the cellular level in animal models, or it may provide prophylactic treatment of poststroke depression, thus improving rehabilitation participation. Important criticisms of the trial include its relatively small sample size and short duration of follow-up. Overall, the FLAME trial represents one of the first studies to demonstrate a pharmacologic effect in improving poststroke recovery.

Question

Does fluoxetine treatment improve motor recovery in patients with acute ischemic stroke and hemiparesis?

Answer

Yes, initiation of fluoxetine treatment in the acute ischemic stroke period, in combination with intensive physiotherapy, safely improves motor recovery.

CHAPTER 17

CAROTID ENDARTERECTOMY FOR ASYMPTOMATIC CAROTID ARTERY STENOSIS

Endarterectomy for Asymptomatic Carotid Artery Stenosis

Executive Committee for the Asymptomatic Carotid Atherosclerosis Study. *JAMA.* 1995;273(18):1421–1428

BACKGROUND

The NASCET trial had shown a benefit in stroke prevention from carotid endarterectomy (CEA) in patients with symptomatic internal carotid artery stenosis. However, prior to the Asymptomatic Carotid Atherosclerosis Study (ACAS), it was unclear whether patients with asymptomatic yet hemodynamically significant carotid stenosis would also benefit from surgery, because at the time these patients had an increased annual stroke rate of 2% to 5%. The ACAS endeavored to answer this question by randomizing patients with 60% or greater carotid stenosis to receive CEA or treatment with aggressive medical therapy alone.

OBJECTIVES

To evaluate whether the addition of CEA to medical therapy would result in improved outcomes in patients with asymptomatic high-grade internal carotid artery stenosis.

METHODS

Prospective, randomized trial conducted at 39 medical centers in the United States and Canada between 1987 and 1993.

Patients

1,659 patients with >60% internal carotid artery stenosis by angiogram within 60 days (or confirmed with ultrasound if angiogram performed >60 days prior) were enrolled if they had no prior cerebrovascular events in the distribution of the stenotic artery. Notable exclusion criteria included history of vertebrobasilar events, contralateral events within the previous 45 days, and contraindications to aspirin.

Interventions

All patients received aspirin 325 mg daily in addition to risk factor modification during the study period. Patients randomized to receive surgery underwent CEA within 2 weeks of randomization.

Outcomes

The primary outcome was initially ipsilateral TIA or cerebral infarction or any perioperative TIA, stroke, or death. Starting in March 2013, this was changed to ipsilateral cerebral infarction or perioperative stroke or death. Outcomes were measured over a median follow-up period of 2.7 years and extrapolated to a predicted 5-year event rate. Secondary outcome analyses included major stroke (resulting in at least moderate–severe disability) and any TIA, stroke, or death.

KEY RESULTS

- 5-year event risk for the initial primary outcome was significantly lower in the surgical group compared to the medical group (8.2% vs. 19.2%, RRR = 0.57, 95% CI = 0.39–0.70, $p < 0.001$).
- 5-year event risk for ipsilateral cerebral infarction or perioperative stroke or death was lower in the surgical group compared to the medical group (5.1% vs. 11.0%, RRR = 0.53, 95% CI = 0.22–0.72, $p = 0.004$).
- There were no significant differences between the groups in any combination of secondary outcomes.

STUDY CONCLUSIONS

In patients with high-grade asymptomatic internal carotid artery stenosis, CEA was associated with a reduction in 5-year ipsilateral ischemic event risk compared to medical therapy alone.

COMMENTARY

The ACAS trial was undertaken to evaluate whether CEA would have a similarly positive effect on stroke prevention in asymptomatic high-grade carotid stenosis patients as it did in those with symptomatic carotid disease. Even when accounting for perioperative complications, the study did show fewer primary outcome events in the CEA group, with Kaplan–Meier curves crossing at around 10 months and showing a significant reduction in the surgical group by 3 years ($p < 0.05$). In contrast to symptomatic carotid studies, however, the results of ACAS showed that certain subpopulations may be more likely to benefit from surgery than others. Specifically, CEA was shown to reduce the 5-year event rate in men by 66% (95% CI = 36%–82%) compared to only 17% in women (95% CI = –96%–65%), and younger patients appeared to derive a greater benefit from surgery, although significant differences between groups were not observed. The later asymptomatic carotid surgery trial (ACST) trial[1] also showed a benefit of CEA in asymptomatic carotid stenosis patients, which was independently effective in men and women, but not in those above the age of 75. Yet there is much doubt about the validity of these conclusions in 2016. From rates of 2% to 5% in the mid-1980s, annual stroke rates in medically treated patients with asymptomatic carotid stenosis had fallen to less than 1% by 2010 (with the exception of those with 70% to 99% stenosis in whom the risk of any stroke, ipsi- or contralateral, approaches 2%). With such low rates in medically treated patients, it is doubtful that surgery could outperform medical therapy. At the time of the ACAS and ACST trials, statin use was not widespread, and that may account in part for the decrease in risk over time. It is notable that a graded effect from CEA that was dependent on patient lipid level was found in ACST. The ongoing CREST-2 trial will independently compare CEA and CAS to intensive MM.

Question

Does CEA reduce the risk of ipsilateral ischemic events in patients with high-grade asymptomatic internal carotid artery stenosis?

Answer

In 2016, the jury is still out. We await the results of the CREST-2 trial to update our knowledge.

Reference

1. Halliday A, Mansfield A, Marro J, et al. Prevention of disabling and fatal strokes by successful carotid endarterectomy in patients without recent neurological symptoms: randomised controlled trial. *Lancet.* 2004;363(9420):1491–1502.

EXTENDED MONITORING FOR PAROXYSMAL ATRIAL FIBRILLATION

Atrial Fibrillation in Patients with Cryptogenic Stroke

Gladstone DJ, Spring M, Dorian P, et al; EMBRACE Investigators and Coordinators. *NEJM*. 2014;370(26):2467–2477

BACKGROUND

Cryptogenic strokes, defined as a stroke or TIA without identified etiology after a standard workup, make up approximately 25% of ischemic strokes. Paroxysmal atrial fibrillation (pAF) is one common cause of stroke that may not be detected with 24 to 48 hours of cardiac arrhythmia monitoring; hence, patients with occult pAF may leave the hospital with a diagnosis of cryptogenic stroke. The motivation for an exhaustive search for pAF as a cause of cryptogenic stroke was based on the efficacy of anticoagulation for secondary stroke prevention. AF represents a highly treatable risk factor for ischemic stroke; with anticoagulant therapy, there is a 64% reduction in risk of stroke and 25% reduction in mortality. At the time of this study, the best approach to detect pAF and the optimal duration of monitoring were unclear.

OBJECTIVES

To evaluate whether prolonged noninvasive ambulatory electrocardiogram (ECG) monitoring would increase the detection of AF in high-risk patients.

METHODS

Open-label, multicenter, RCT at 16 Canadian centers from 2009 through 2012.

Patients

572 patients 55 years of age or older without known AF and an ischemic stroke or TIA of undetermined etiology within the past 6 months were randomized. Standard workup comprised 12-lead ECG, ambulatory ECG monitoring for at least 24 hours, echocardiography, and brain and neurovascular imaging. Patients were excluded if stroke type was determined to be small-vessel or large-vessel disease.

Interventions

Intervention group involved ambulatory ECG monitoring with a 30-day event-triggered loop recorder. The patients in the control group completed one additional 24-hour Holter study.

Outcomes

The primary outcome was the detection of one or more episodes of ECG-documented AF or atrial flutter exceeding 30 seconds within 90 days from randomization. Secondary outcomes included institution of oral anticoagulant at 90 days, AF of any duration, and adherence to monitoring.

KEY RESULTS

- AF lasting 30 seconds or longer was detected in 16.1% of the intervention group as compared to 3.2% of the control group (number needed to screen 8, 95% CI = 5.7–12.5, $p < 0.001$).
- AF of any duration detected was 19.7% in the intervention group and 4.7% in the control group (number needed to screen 7, 95% CI = 4.9–10.2, $p < 0.001$).
- At 90 days, 18.6% of the intervention group and 11.1% of the control group were treated with anticoagulants (95% CI = 1.6–13.3, $p = 0.01$).

STUDY CONCLUSIONS

Ambulatory ECG monitoring for 30 days detected AF in one in six patients with cryptogenic stroke and was superior to an additional round of 24-hour ECG monitoring.

COMMENTARY

The EMBRACE trial was performed to evaluate whether extended cardiac monitoring was technically feasible and whether it improved detection of pAF in patients with cryptogenic stroke. The landmark findings in this trial were that extended cardiac monitoring significantly increased the detection rate of pAF and altered therapies for secondary stroke prevention. CRYSTAL-AF supported these findings by showing that with an implantable device allowing for extended periods of continuous ECG monitoring, the detection of AF increased with longer duration of monitoring (8.9% at 6 months vs. 30% at 3 years). These two trials shifted the clinical practice to the routine pursuit of extended cardiac monitoring for cryptogenic stroke and consideration for implantable loop recorder placement if strong clinical suspicion of pAF exists.

Question

Should extended ambulatory cardiac monitoring be performed in patients with cryptogenic stroke?

Answer

Yes, for patients with cryptogenic stroke, despite unrevealing inpatient or 24-to-48-hour ambulatory cardiac monitoring, extended ambulatory cardiac monitoring for at least 30 days is warranted.

CHAPTER 19

THE NATIONAL INSTITUTES OF HEALTH STROKE SCALE

Measurements of Acute Cerebral Infarction: A Clinical Examination Scale

Brott T, Adams HP Jr, Olinger CP, et al. *Stroke*. 1989;20(7):864–870

BACKGROUND

Some acute stroke management decisions depend on the clinical severity of the cerebral infarction. However, prior to the National Institutes of Health Stroke Scale (NIHSS), systems for clinical assessment had not been appropriately validated for interexaminer reliability or correlation with the extent and location of the infarction. The NIHSS was developed in order to provide clinicians with a brief but comprehensive neurologic examination scale that was reliable between practitioners and valid when correlated with brain imaging and clinical outcome measures.

OBJECTIVES

To develop a neurologic examination scale for the accurate assessment of acute ischemic stroke severity.

METHODS

Reliability and validity trial of a clinical assessment scale with field testing conducted at two US medical centers in 1984 and 1985.

Patients

For design of the examination format, 10 patients with ischemic stroke within 3 weeks were enrolled. For assessing stroke scale reliability, 24 patients with ischemic stroke within 1 week were enrolled. To test validity, use of the stroke scale in a therapy trial (naloxone for acute ischemic stroke) included 65 patients with ischemic stroke within 48 hours.

Interventions

Scale items were obtained from four existing assessment forms—the Toronto Stroke Scale, Oxbury Initial Severity Scale, Cincinnati Stroke Scale, and Edinburgh-2 Coma Scale—as well as from discussion with investigators participating in the National Institute of Neurological Disorders and Stroke (NINDS) treatment studies. Scale components included neurologic signs correlating with the distribution of each of the major cerebral arteries, as well as with overall dysfunction. Scale item grade differences were designed to be as clear as possible.

Outcomes

Scale items were evaluated individually. Test reliability was analyzed using the kappa (κ) statistic to determine interrater reliability. Neurologic examination was performed twice by a staff neurologist and observed by a neurology house officer, neurology nurse, and emergency room nurse, and reliability was assessed both among clinicians and from first to second examination. Validity was assessed through the correlation of scale scores with volume of infarction on head CT and with three different measures of functional outcome at 3 months.

KEY RESULTS
- The scale was applied quickly (mean 6.6 ± 1.3 minutes) in all patients. A mean of 1.3 items (out of 15) could not be scored.
- Interrater reliability was high, with mean $\kappa = 0.69$ (perfect agreement = 1.00, perfect disagreement = −1.00). Test–retest reliability was high (mean $\kappa = 0.66$–0.77) and correlation between the first and second examination was 0.98 ($p < 0.0001$).
- Correlation between initial scale score and CT infarct volume at 1 week was 0.78 ($p = 0.0001$).
- Correlation between initial scale score and functional outcome at 3 months was 0.53 ($p = 0.0001$).

STUDY CONCLUSIONS
The NIHSS is a reliable, valid, and easily applied clinical assessment tool for quantifying acute ischemic stroke severity.

COMMENTARY

The NIHSS study was undertaken to evaluate whether the neurologic examination scale was effective in quantifying acute ischemic stroke severity. The importance of having such a validated and universally accepted assessment tool cannot be overstated, both for clinical decision-making and for testing new stroke treatments. The NIHSS was found to be reliable, valid, quick, and practical, thus making it an ideal measure with independently confirmed reliability.[1] The scale has subsequently undergone minor adjustments, specifically the removal of pupillary response and plantar reflex, to further enhance validity. It is now the most commonly used assessment scale in stroke treatment trials and clinical practice worldwide for determining patient eligibility for acute therapies, such as IV tPA and intra-arterial interventions.

Question
Is the NIHSS a valid predictor of acute ischemic stroke severity?

Answer
Yes, the NIHSS was designed and tested for its internal and external validity, precision, and discrimination and can be applied expediently for the quantification of stroke severity.

Reference
1. Goldstein LB, Bertels C, Davis JN. Interrater reliability of the NIH stroke scale. *Arch Neurol.* 1989;46(6):660–662.

CEREBRAL HEMORRHAGE

SECTION 2

Steven M. Greenberg ■ David J. Lin ■ Saad Mir

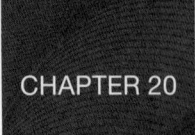

CHAPTER 20

BLOOD PRESSURE REGULATION IN PARENCHYMAL INTRACEREBRAL HEMORRHAGE

Rapid Blood-Pressure Lowering in Patients with Acute Intracerebral Hemorrhage

Anderson CS, Heeley E, Huang Y, et al. INTERACT 2 trial. *NEJM*. 2013;368(25):2355–2365

BACKGROUND

Intracerebral hemorrhage (ICH) constitutes 10% to 15% of all strokes and has very high morbidity and mortality rates. Despite this, ICH therapies remain minimal aside from blood pressure control because hypertension portends worse outcomes. Clinical practice varied greatly, and it was unclear if intensive blood pressure reduction was beneficial or safe in comparison to standard blood pressure reduction. In 2008, the INTERACT trial demonstrated that intensive blood pressure reduction (systolic <140 mm Hg) in acute ICH reduced hematoma growth more effectively and safely than standard of care (systolic <180 mm Hg). However, the effect of intensive blood pressure reduction on long-term clinical outcomes remained unclear, thus prompting the INTERACT 2 trial.

OBJECTIVES

To determine if intensive, acute blood pressure control improves functional outcomes in ICH patients.

METHODS

Prospective, randomized, open-treatment, blinded end-point trial involving 144 hospitals in 21 countries.

Patients

2,839 patients with ICH were randomized to receive early intensive blood pressure control (*n* = 1,403) with target systolic level <140 mm Hg or guideline-recommended treatment (*n* = 1,436) of a target systolic level of <180 mm Hg. Exclusion criteria included structural causes of the bleed, coma, massive bleed with poor prognosis, or if surgery was planned.

Interventions

Early intensive blood pressure control within 6 hours vs. guideline-recommended blood pressure control.

Outcomes

The primary outcome was death or major disability as defined by a score of 3 to 6 on the modified Rankin scale (mRS) at 3 months. Ordinal analysis of the primary outcome was utilized to assess shift toward better mRS scores.

KEY RESULTS

• No significant difference in proportion of patients with death or major disability at 3 months in intensive treatment group vs. guideline treatment (52% vs. 55.6%, OR = 0.87, 95% CI = 0.75–1.01, p = 0.06).
• Ordinal analysis showed a favorable shift in the distribution of scores on the mRS with the intensive blood pressure reduction arm (pooled OR = 0.87, 95% CI = 0.77–1.00, p = 0.04).
• Significantly less problems and improved overall health quality at 90 days in intensive treatment group based on the EuroQoL five dimensions questionnaire for health status (mean ± SD utility score, 0.60 ± 0.39 vs. 0.55 ± 0.40, p = 0.002).
• No significant difference in hematoma growth between the groups after 24 hours (relative difference, 4.5%, 95% CI = −3.1–12.7, p = 0.27).

STUDY CONCLUSIONS

Intensive blood pressure reduction in acute ICH does not reduce rate of death or significant morbidity, but does cause a favorable shift toward improved functional outcomes.

COMMENTARY

Because only 20% of ICH survivors are independent at 6 months, treatment strategies that can reduce morbidity are paramount. Nonrandomized data suggest that lower blood pressure goals are associated with better outcomes, which was safely validated in the pilot INTERACT trial. The subsequent INTERACT 2 showed that intensive blood pressure reduction can shift toward improved functional outcomes, suggesting a potential impact on alleviating healthcare. Limitations of the study included shorter times from ICH to treatment and shorter times from randomization to treatment in the intensive group. This may have overestimated the effect of intensive treatment, because early reduction may be more beneficial than absolute reduction in pressure. Moreover, absence of standardized blood pressure reduction regimens may have led to various drug class utilizations with unknown effects on clinical outcomes.

Question

Is intensive lowering of blood pressure in acute ICH beneficial for patients?

Answer

Possibly. Intensive blood pressure reduction (systolic <140 mm Hg) shifts patients toward better outcomes, though further studies will be needed to reproduce these findings and demonstrate long-term benefits.

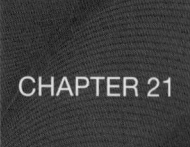

CHAPTER 21

EARLY SURGERY FOR SPONTANEOUS INTRACEREBRAL HEMORRHAGE AND HYDROCEPHALUS

Early Surgery versus Initial Conservative Treatment in Patients with Spontaneous Supratentorial Intracerebral Haematomas in the International Surgical Trial in Intracerebral Haemorrhage (STICH): A Randomised Trial

Mendelow AD, Gregson BA, Fernandes HM, et al; STICH Trial Investigators. *Lancet.* 2005;365:387–397

BACKGROUND

Surgical evacuation of ICH hematomas has been practiced since the mid-1900s. Though, prior to 2005, several studies suggested conflicting benefit, which led to variability in patient selection and surgical approaches, the STICH trial was the first modern study to assess long-term functional outcomes in patients randomized to hematoma evacuation.

OBJECTIVES

To determine whether early surgical evacuation of spontaneous supratentorial ICH confers any long-term benefit over initial MM.

METHODS

Prospective, randomized, open treatment, parallel-group trial involving 83 hospitals in 27 countries.

Patients

1,033 patients with spontaneous supratentorial ICH were randomized to early surgery ($n = 503$) or conservative treatment ($n = 530$). Surgery had to be of uncertain benefit and initiated within 24 hours of randomization. Exclusion criteria included severe disability prior to the ICH and bleeds due to aneurysm, AVMs, tumors, or trauma. Infratentorial ICH and extension into brainstem were also excluded.

Interventions

Early surgical evacuation of supratentorial ICH within 72 hours of onset and within 24 hours of randomization vs. MM.

Outcomes

Glasgow Coma Scale (GCS) obtained by postal questionnaires sent directly to patients at 6 months follow-up. Secondary outcomes included mortality, Barthel index, and modified Rankin scale (mRS).

KEY RESULTS
- 26% of the medical group ultimately had surgery.
- No difference in extended GCS, Barthel indices, mRS, or 6-month mortality in surgical group compared to medical group.
- Early surgery had more favorable outcomes if ICH was ≤1 cm from cortical surface (absolute benefit 8%, $p = 0.02$).

STUDY CONCLUSIONS
Early surgical evacuation of ICH is not likely to confer morbidity or mortality benefit over conservative MM.

COMMENTARY

This trial demonstrated nonsuperiority from early surgical hematoma evacuation in acute ICH compared to initial medical treatment, though a quarter of patients randomized to the medical group ultimately did require surgery. This likely supports surgical management for severe circumstances, such as a patient who may be failing medical therapy or with impending herniation. Subgroup analysis demonstrated a potential benefit in surgical evacuation of superficial cortical bleeds. These findings prompted the STICH II trial, which also supported no clinical benefit in early surgical evacuation of hematomas compared to initial MM. Despite its strength, the STICH trial used dichotomized functional outcomes and thus may have missed shifts toward better outcomes if an ordinal outcome had been used.

Question
Does early surgical evacuation confer long-term benefit over initial MM in patients with ICH?

Answer
No, MM is not inferior to early surgical evacuation of ICH with regard to long-term outcomes.

CHAPTER 22

AVOIDANCE OF LONG-TERM ANTICOAGULATION FOR ATRIAL FIBRILLATION AFTER INTRACEREBRAL HEMORRHAGE

Can Patients be Anticoagulated after Intracerebral Hemorrhage?
Eckman MH, Rosand J, Knudsen K, et al. *Stroke.* 2003;34:1710–1716

BACKGROUND
The annual risk of recurrent ICH in patients with a history of ICH can be as high as 10% to 15%. Anticoagulation significantly increases this risk, creating a difficult clinical scenario when ICH patients also have AF or mechanical valves. A decision analysis was created to model the effects of anticoagulation in patients with a history of ICH given ethical concerns of randomizing patients to a potentially harmful intervention.

OBJECTIVES
To determine whether withholding anticoagulation for stroke prevention in the setting of AF confers morbidity or mortality benefit in patients with a prior history of ICH.

METHODS
Markov state transition decision model stratified by location of hemorrhage (lobar vs. deep) with outcomes measured in quality-adjusted life years (QALYs).

Assumptions
- For patients not receiving anticoagulation, any embolic stroke that led to anticoagulation indefinitely with fixed 3-month morbidity score of neurologic function.
- For patients receiving anticoagulation, ICH or subdural hematoma that led to indefinite cessation of anticoagulation with 3-month fixed morbidity score of neurologic function.
- Quality adjustment factors after embolic stroke were correlated to Glasgow Outcome Scores used in ICH.
- Annual risk for recurrent ICH with a history of lobar ICH was set at 15%. Annual risk for recurrent ICH with a history of deep ICH was set at 2.1%.
- Annual risk for embolic stroke from AF was set at 4.5%, with warfarin reducing this risk by 68%.

Interventions
Simulated initiation or withholding of anticoagulation in patients with a history of ICH.

Outcomes
Quality-adjusted life years (QALYs).

KEY RESULTS

- For patients with a history of lobar ICH, withholding anticoagulation resulted in 1.9 more QALYs compared to anticoagulation (5.4 vs. 3.5, respectively). This finding was consistent in subsequent sensitivity analyses by varying the parameters for risk of embolism and risk of recurrent ICH.
- For patients with history of deep ICH, both withholding and initiating anticoagulation had similar QALYs (7.8 vs. 7.5, respectively). Anticoagulation was preferred when the annual rate of recurrent ICH was 1.4%, or the annual risk of ischemic stroke was 6.5%/yr.

STUDY CONCLUSIONS

For patients with a history of lobar ICH who also need anticoagulation, the risk of recurrent ICH likely outweighs the benefit of reducing embolic stroke risk. For patients with a history of deep ICH, the risk of recurrent ICH from anticoagulation may be outweighed if the annual thromboembolic risk is high.

COMMENTARY

Prior to this decision analysis, clinicians were faced with complex management decisions of patients with a history of ICH and indications for anticoagulation with unclear risks. The findings suggest that the risk of recurrent ICH likely outweighs the benefits of anticoagulation. Although not randomized data, the analyses used peer-reviewed literature and exhaustive modeling with varying assumptions to assess for confidence in the primary findings. Whereas a standard 4.5% was used in modeling annual stroke risk, sensitivity analyses modeled up to 20% annual stroke risk to avoid underestimation. One caveat is the generalizability of these results in an era with newer oral anticoagulants. For example, in 2011 the ARISTOTLE trial demonstrated that apixaban had significantly fewer strokes and reduced ICH risk compared to warfarin, and thus the risk of recurrent ICH would also be different with oral anticoagulants.

Question

Should a patient with lobar ICH and AF be anticoagulated with warfarin for ischemic stroke prophylaxis?

Answer

No, indefinite warfarin is predicted to confer more morbidity and mortality from recurrent ICH in patients with a history of lobar ICH.

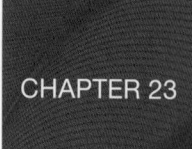

NIMODIPINE FOR PREVENTION OF DELAYED NEUROLOGIC INJURY AFTER SUBARACHNOID HEMORRHAGE

CHAPTER 23

Cerebral Arterial Spasm—A Controlled Trial of Nimodipine in Patients with Subarachnoid Hemorrhage

Allen GS, Ahn HS, Preziosi TJ. *N Engl J Med*. 1983;308(11):619–624

BACKGROUND

Delayed cerebral ischemia (previously referred to as vasospasm) is a known complication of subarachnoid hemorrhage and leads to ischemic stroke and secondary neurologic deficits. Previous studies in animals have suggested that nimodipine inhibits cerebral arterial contraction and may prevent or reduce the severity of vasospasm. This is the first large trial in humans to determine whether nimodipine would prevent or reduce the severity of ischemic neurologic deficits from delayed arterial spasm after aneurysmal subarachnoid hemorrhage.

OBJECTIVES

To test the effectiveness of nimodipine in preventing or altering the severity of ischemic neurologic deficits because of vasospasm after aneurysmal subarachnoid hemorrhage.

METHODS

Prospective, randomized, double-blind, placebo-controlled trial of 125 neurologically normal patients with intracranial aneurysms and subarachnoid hemorrhages at five university centers between 1979 and 1982.

Patients

Inclusion criteria included a normal neurologic examination, demonstration of subarachnoid hemorrhage on CT scan within 96 hours of starting the study medication, and demonstration of an intracranial aneurysm by angiography. Notable caveats that could still be present in a "normal" neurologic examination included stiff neck, headache, fever, photophobia, drowsiness, and isolated cranial nerve palsies.

Interventions

Patients were randomized in a double-blind manner to either nimodipine or placebo for a 21-day treatment period.

Outcomes

The primary outcomes were development of a neurologic deficit from cerebral arterial spasm and severity of the deficit at the end of the treatment period. Secondary outcomes included the degree of vasospasm on the cerebral angiograms and the amount of basal subarachnoid hemorrhage on CT scans.

KEY RESULTS

- 1 of 56 patients given nimodipine vs. 8 of 60 patients given placebo developed a neurologic deficit from cerebral arterial spasm that persisted and was severe or caused death by the end of the 21-day treatment period ($p = 0.03$, Fisher's exact test).
- An increase in subarachnoid blood was not associated with worse neurologic outcome among patients who received nimodipine, whereas it was in patients given placebo.
- The overall rate of aneurysmal rebleeding was similar in the two treatment groups.
- There were no reported side effects from nimodipine.

STUDY CONCLUSIONS

Nimodipine should be given to patients who are neurologically normal after subarachnoid hemorrhage in order to reduce the occurrence of severe neurologic deficits because of delayed cerebral arterial spasm.

COMMENTARY

Vasospasm after subarachnoid hemorrhage resulting in ischemic stroke is a major cause of morbidity and mortality. Nimodipine, a calcium channel blocker that crosses the blood–brain barrier, had some preclinical evidence to suggest that it might selectively block cerebral arterial smooth muscle cells to prevent vasospasm. This was the first well-powered trial in humans to test the efficacy of nimodipine for preventing vasospasm after aneurysmal subarachnoid hemorrhage. The results of the study were encouraging, showing that patients given nimodipine after aneurysmal subarachnoid hemorrhage had better neurologic outcome as compared to placebo. One major caveat to the study is that included patients did not have major neurologic deficits at the time that they were started on nimodipine, a criterion that would be difficult to achieve in clinical practice given that many patients present to hospitals with neurologic deficits from subarachnoid hemorrhage. The idea that nimodipine improves neurologic outcomes after subarachnoid hemorrhage has held up in more recent trials and meta-analyses. However, nimodipine has not been shown to have a major effect on angiographic vasospasm (when directly measuring arterial diameter), arguing that the effects of nimodipine may involve broader neuroprotective mechanisms.

Question

Does nimodipine reduce severity of neurologic deficits after subarachnoid hemorrhage?

Answer

Yes, nimodipine appears to reduce the severity of neurologic deficits as a result of cerebral arterial spasm after aneurysmal subarachnoid hemorrhage and should be given to all patients presenting with aneurysmal subarachnoid hemorrhage.

CHAPTER 24

INFERIORITY OF SURGICAL RESECTION TO MEDICAL MANAGEMENT OF UNRUPTURED AVM

Medical Management with or without Interventional Therapy for Unruptured Brain Arteriovenous Malformations (ARUBA): A Multicentre, Non-blinded, Randomised Trial

Mohr JP, Parides MK, Stapf C, et al; ARUBA Investigators. *Lancet.* 2014;383:614–621

BACKGROUND

With advancements in imaging, discovery of unruptured arteriovenous malformations (AVMs) has doubled over the past few decades. Rupture rates for AVMs range from about 1% to 4% annually depending on grade. Prior to 2014, management of unruptured AVMs varied greatly because of difference in perceived rupture risk and intervention safety. As a result, it was unclear whether MM was superior or inferior to interventional treatments to prevent AVM rupture.

OBJECTIVES

To determine risk of stroke or death in patients with unruptured AVMs who were treated medically with or without interventional therapy.

METHODS

Prospective, parallel design, nonblinded, RCT involving 39 active clinical sites in nine countries.

Patients

226 patients found to have unruptured AVMs amenable to intervention were randomized to either MM ($n = 109$) or MM with interventional treatment ($n = 114$). Exclusion criteria included age <18 years, previous hemorrhage, or AVM not amenable to intervention.

Interventions

Medical management at discretion of physicians (e.g., blood pressure control, seizure control, avoidance of blood thinners) vs. intervention at discretion of physician. Interventions included standard neurosurgery, radiotherapy, embolization, or combination of approaches.

Outcomes

The primary outcome was composite risk of stroke or death, whereas secondary outcome was composite risk of death or neurologic disability (modified Rankin scale score ≥ 2).

KEY RESULTS

- Study stopped early because of superiority of the medical group. Mean follow-up at time of study termination was 33 months.

- Significantly lower risk of stroke or death in medical group compared to interventional group (10.1% vs. 30.7%, RR = 0.33, 95% CI = 0.18–0.61).
- Significantly lower risk of death or neurologic disability in the medical group compared to interventional group (15.1% vs. 46.2%, RR = 0.33, 95% CI = 0.16–0.66).
- No differences in demographics, clinical presentations, Spetzler–Martin grades, and modified Rankin scales. Overall, 62% had Spetzler–Martin grades <2 and no patient had grade >4.
- More patients with preexisting focal deficits and AVM <3 cm in interventional group.

STUDY CONCLUSIONS

For unruptured AVMs, MM alone is superior to MM with intervention in preventing stroke, death, and neurologic disability at least 3 years after treatment.

COMMENTARY

Prior to the ARUBA trial, treatment approaches for unruptured AVMs varied, and related expense estimates for early intervention ranged from $150 to $300 million dollars per year. These findings helped codify a safer and more cost-effective approach to treating unruptured AVMs. The study ended early because of increased treatment risk, raising concerns of potentially missing long-term bleeding risk of medically treated AVMs. However, a recent 5-year follow-up of this trial corroborates the findings favoring medical treatment of AVMs. The study also excluded AVMs that have a substantially higher rupture risk, which have higher risk of rebleeding (4% to 8%) and would therefore be more amenable to intervention instead of MM. Finally, there were no consensus guidelines for intervention approaches that could lead to inconsistencies, higher complication rates, and confounding by indication.

Question

Is medical management alone for unruptured AVMs superior to MM with interventional therapies?

Answer

Yes, for low-grade unruptured AVMs that have not historically bled and are amenable to intervention, medical treatment alone results in reduced risk of stroke, death, and neurologic disability.

CHAPTER 25

PROGNOSTICATION FOR INTRACEREBRAL HEMORRHAGE

The ICH Score: A Simple, Reliable Grading Scale for Intracerebral Hemorrhage

Hemphill JC, Bonovich DC, Besmeritis L, et al. *Stroke*. 2001;32(4):891–897

BACKGROUND

Prior to 2001, predictive outcome scores for ICH were complex and necessitated nuanced knowledge of clinical and radiographic variables. There was a need for a simple yet valid method of predicting outcomes in ICH for clinical care and research.

OBJECTIVES

To create a clinical outcome scale for ICH patients that can be rapidly and reliably implemented.

METHODS

Retrospective, single-center review of all ICH patients admitted in 1 year. Multivariate logistic regression analyses were performed on outcomes, with 30-day mortality as the dependent variable. An outcome risk stratification scale was developed and points were allocated to each variable depending on the strength of the association.

Patients

152 patients who presented to a university hospital with ICH from 1997 to 1998.

KEY RESULTS

- In multivariate analysis, associations with 30-day mortality were significant with GCS score ($p < 0.001$), ICH volume ($p = 0.047$), infratentorial location ($p = 0.03$), age $\geq$80 years ($p = 0.001$), and presence of intraventricular hemorrhage (IVH) ($p = 0.052$).
- ICH score: score from 0 to 6 comprised the following:
  - GCS score: 3 to 4 (2 pt), 5 to 12 (1 pt), 13 to 15 (0 pt)
  - ICH volume: $\geq$30 cm^3 (1 pt), <30 cm^3 (0 pt)
  - IVH present: Yes (1 pt), No (0 pt)
  - Infratentorial: Yes (1 pt), No (0 pt)
  - Age: $\geq$80 years (1 pt), <80 years (0 pt)
- ICH score patient distribution: 0 (17%), 1 (21%), 2 (18%), 3 (21%), 4 (19%), 5 (4%), 6 (0%).
- 30-Day mortality rates for patients with ICH scores of 1, 2, 3, 4, and 5 were 13%, 26%, 72%, 97%, and 100%, respectively. No patient scored 6.

STUDY CONCLUSIONS

The ICH score is simple and is able to reliably estimate 30-day mortality in patients with ICH.

COMMENTARY

The ICH score allows health care providers to easily quantify neurologic injury severity and estimate 30-day mortality, thereby facilitating treatment decisions and research studies. The score's strength is highlighted by its weight on GCS being divided into three strata, which is most associated with 30-day mortality. Previous score predictors dichotomized GCS to favorable (<8) or unfavorable (>8), which may miss clinically significant transitions in GCS. However, in an attempt to maintain simplicity, the score does not incorporate other prognostic variables that may have an influence on risk of 30-day mortality. As a result, the authors emphasize that the score is not intended as a codified mortality tool, but an estimate for clinical trajectory of patients. The score also does not account for patients for whom treatment may have been withdrawn, which may create self-fulfilling prophecies for poor outcomes with certain ICH scores. Similarly, the study is limited to 30-day outcomes and is not validated for long-term prognosis. The ICH score was later externally and independently validated, thus promoting its use in treatment protocols and clinical studies.

Question

Can ICH patients be simply and reliably stratified by risk of mortality with any clinical scoring tool?

Answer

Yes, the ICH score is a 6-point scale predictive of disease severity and 30-day short-term mortality risk.

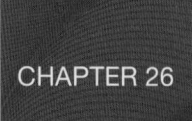

CHAPTER 26

ACUTE ENDOVASCULAR TREATMENT FOR RUPTURED SUBARACHNOID HEMORRHAGE

Joel Salinas ■ Ayush Batra

Aneurysmal SAH in Patients with Hunt and Hess Grade 4 or 5: Treatment Using the Guglielmi Detachable Coil System

Weir RU, Marcellus ML, Do HM, et al. *AJNR Am J Neuroradiol*. 2003;24:585–590

BACKGROUND

Patients with poor grade (Hunt and Hess grade 4 or 5) subarachnoid hemorrhage (SAH) after aneurysmal rupture have high morbidity and mortality rates and were often excluded from early aggressive treatment. This retrospective study assessed the outcome of poor grade patients who were treated with early aggressive endovascular treatment using Guglielmi detachable coil (GDC) embolization.

OBJECTIVES

To determine morbidity and mortality of poor grade aneurysmal SAH patients who are treated with early GDC embolization.

METHODS

Retrospective, single-center review of patients from 1994 to 2001.

Patients

Twenty-seven consecutive Hunt and Hess grade 4 or 5 aneurysmal SAH patients who presented to a single center and were treated with GDC embolization. All patients were treated within 72 hours of SAH onset. Decision to treat with endovascular therapy was based on joint neurosurgical and interventional neuroradiology assessment of aneurysm morphology, which was judged to be conducive for complete or near-complete occlusion.

Interventions

Endovascular GDC embolization with the goal of complete aneurysm thrombosis, though in some cases coil embolization partially occluded the aneurysm to prevent acute rebleeding of the dome.

Outcomes

Primary outcome was survival at short-term follow-up (30 days) and modified Rankin scale at long-term follow-up for survivors. Secondary outcomes included percentage aneurysm occlusion after embolization, perioperative complications, and symptoms of vasospasm.

KEY RESULTS

- 16 (59%) patients died within 30 days of SAH, whereas 8 (30%) had a good clinical outcome at mean long-term follow-up of 23 months (range 6 to 44 months).

- One technical (4%) and one clinical (4%) complication occurred at embolization.
- No rebleeding occurred in any of the patients during long-term follow-up. 25 (92%) had vasospasm and 7 required additional endovascular treatment because of worsening clinical status.

STUDY CONCLUSIONS

Comparable to published early aggressive surgical treatment literature, poor grade aneurysmal SAH patients can successfully undergo partial or complete coil embolization despite poor clinical condition and high frequency of perioperative vasospasm, though morbidity and mortality rates remain high in this population.

COMMENTARY

Acute endovascular treatment was not routinely offered in poor grade (Hunt and Hess grade 4 or 5) aneurysmal SAH patients, and most poor grade patients were left out of early aggressive surgical treatment studies because of their high morbidity. This study compared the morbidity and mortality rates in this population to aggressively managed surgical treatments. The findings were further supported by a subsequent retrospective study of 45 similar consecutive patients with 6-month follow-up after treatment with coiling, which demonstrated that about half of the patients had favorable outcomes.[1] However, because the main prognostic factor for poor outcome is likely SAH-related parenchymal damage and delayed cerebral ischemia, these studies suggest that preventing recurrent hemorrhage addresses a single cause of poor outcomes. Selection bias of patients who would benefit from aneurysm coiling would therefore have a high chance of influencing the observation of better outcomes in treatment groups. Thus, these two studies influenced practice mostly by reinforcing that poor grade aneurysmal SAH patients could be treated by acute endovascular treatment or early aggressive surgical treatment.

Question

Can patients with poor grade aneurysmal SAH be treated with endovascular coil embolization?

Answer

Yes, poor grade aneurysmal SAH patients may benefit from successful coil embolization despite poor clinical condition and high rate of vasospasm at the time of treatment.

Reference

1. Bergui M, Bradac GB. Acute endovascular treatment of ruptured aneurysm in poor-grade patients. *Neuroradiology.* 2004;46(2):161–164.

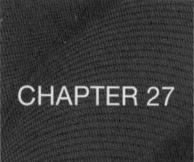

NEUROSURGICAL CLIPPING VS. ENDOVASCULAR COILING OF RUPTURED INTRACRANIAL ANEURYSMS

CHAPTER 27

Ayush Batra ■ Joel Salinas

International Subarachnoid Aneurysm Trial (ISAT) of Neurosurgical Clipping versus Endovascular Coiling in 2143 Patients with Ruptured Intracranial Aneurysms: A Randomized Trial

Molyneux AJ; the ISAT Collaborative Group. *Lancet.* 2002;360:1267–1274

BACKGROUND

At the time of this trial, endovascular coil embolization was becoming used more frequently as an alternative to surgical craniotomy and clipping for treatment of ruptured aneurysmal subarachnoid hemorrhage (SAH). This multicenter randomized trial sought to compare safety and efficacy of endovascular coiling to neurosurgical clipping in aneurysms deemed suitable to either treatment.

OBJECTIVES

To determine morbidity and mortality of aneurysmal SAH patients treated with endovascular coiling compared to those treated with surgical clipping.

METHODS

Randomized, multicenter trial with per-protocol analysis from 1994 to 1999.

Patients

2,143 patients were enrolled with aneurysmal SAH. Participants were eligible if they had a definite aneurysmal SAH proven by imaging or lumbar puncture within 28 days and were judged by the neurosurgeon and interventional neuroradiologist that angiographic anatomy was amenable to either intervention, but with uncertainty about which of the two treatments was indicated.

Interventions

Patients were randomly assigned to either neurosurgical clipping ($n = 1,070$) or endovascular treatment via detachable platinum coil embolization ($n = 1,073$).

Outcomes

Primary outcome was proportion of patients with modified Rankin scale (mRS) indicating dependency or death (score 3 to 6) after 1 year. Clinical outcomes were assessed at 2 months and at 1 year.

KEY RESULTS

- 190/801 (23.7%) of endovascular patients were dependent or dead after 1 year compared to 243/793 (30.6%) of neurosurgical clipping patients.

- Relative and absolute risk of endovascular treatment vs. neurosurgical clipping was 22.6% (95% CI = 8.9–34.2) and 6.9% (95% CI = 2.5–11.3), respectively.
- Recurrent hemorrhage incidence at 1 year was 2 per 1,275 patient-years for endovascular treatment and 0 per 1,081 patient-years for neurosurgical treatment.

STUDY CONCLUSIONS

Aneurysmal SAH patients who are amenable with uncertain benefit to either endovascular coil embolization or neurosurgical clipping are more likely to have disability-free survival at 1 year with endovascular treatment compared to clipping. Although rebleeding risk is slightly lower in neurosurgical clipping compared to coil embolization after 1 year, the risk is relatively low in both treatments.

COMMENTARY

This multicenter randomized trial helped to assess the relative safety and efficacy of endovascular treatment compared to neurosurgical clipping in aneurysmal rupture where angiographic anatomy would be amenable to either treatment, but benefit was uncertain between the two options. Trial recruitment was halted early, with findings at 1 year demonstrating the reduction in relative risk of dependence or death in the endovascular treatment group. Subsequent results supported that the early survival advantage of those treated with endovascular treatment continued in follow-up through 18 years.[1] Other secondary outcomes were also considered in the follow-up study, including risk of epilepsy in follow-up after SAH, which was significantly lower in the endovascular group. Risk of rebleeding after 1 year remained higher in the endovascular group compared to neurosurgical clipping, but the overall risk remained low.

Question

Should patients with aneurysmal SAH who have angiographic anatomy amenable to neurosurgical clipping or endovascular therapy be preferentially treated with coil embolization?

Answer

Yes, aneurysmal SAH patients who undergo endovascular coil embolization have better long-term disability-free survival compared to neurosurgical clipping.

Reference

1. Molyneaux AJ, Birks J, Clarke A, et al. The durability of endovascular coiling versus neurosurgical clipping of ruptured cerebral aneurysm: 18 year follow-up of the UK cohort of the International Subarachnoid Aneurysm Trial (ISAT). *Lancet*. 2015;385(9969):691–697.

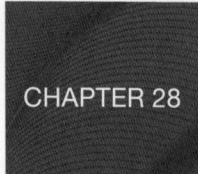

CHAPTER 28	WITHDRAWAL OF SUPPORT IN INTRACEREBRAL HEMORRHAGE BECAUSE OF PREDICTED POOR PROGNOSIS MAY LEAD TO SELF-FULFILLING PROPHECY

Withdrawal of Support in Intracerebral Hemorrhage May Lead to Self-fulfilling Prophecies

Becker KJ, Baxter AB, Cohen WA, et al. *Neurology*. 2001;56(6):766–772

BACKGROUND

Clinical examination and radiographic findings are the primary components of predictive outcome scores for ICH. However, the morbidity and mortality data from which these scores were derived allowed inclusion of patients who had withdrawal of medical support. As a result, poor predictive scores may overestimate true mortality, leading to withdrawal of care and subsequent death and thus to a "self-fulfilling prophecy"; yet, the clinical course of these patients may be different if given maximal medical therapy.

OBJECTIVES

To determine how withdrawal of care and surgical intervention affect prognostic models in ICH patients and to evaluate attitudes about futility of care among neurologists and neurosurgeons.

METHODS

Retrospective, single-center review of all supratentorial ICH patients in a 3-year span. Univariate and multivariate analyses were done to assess effects of radiography, clinical variables, surgical intervention, and withdrawal of care on in-hospital mortality. Also, neurology and neurosurgery physicians involved in direct care of ICH patients were surveyed anonymously regarding cases, with variables assessed in the analysis. They were asked to opine if patients should receive decompressive surgery, surgery if deterioration, aggressive medical care only, or withdraw support. These responses were compared to the historical outcomes of the patients.

Patients

Eighty-seven patients who presented with supratentorial ICH to a single center from 1994 to 1997. Exclusion criteria included history of trauma, tumor, subarachnoid bleed, or aneurysm.

Outcomes

Primary outcomes included in-hospital mortality, surgical intervention, and the decision to withdraw medical support.

KEY RESULTS

- Initial GCS score was the only independent predictor of death in multivariate analyses, with all radiographic and clinical variables available at admission (OR, 1.23 per point decrease, 95% CI = 1.02–1.48, p = 0.03).

- Mass effect, lack of surgery, and midline shift were all associated with increased risk of mortality if surgery was employed.
- Older age, midline shift, and left hemisphere ICH all independently predicted absence of surgical intervention.
- Withdrawal of medical care was most predictive of mortality compared to other variables.
- Median length of stay for patients who had care withdrawn was 2 days.
- Physicians tended to underestimate functional recovery in patients presenting with severe neurologic injury.

STUDY CONCLUSIONS

ICH patients with poor predictive scores can have meaningful recovery with maximal medical care. Decisions to withdraw care based on these scores are prevalent among care providers and may perpetuate self-fulfilling prophecies.

COMMENTARY

Predictive scores can help triage treatment and research, but they can also lead to aggregated cohort-level outcomes being projected to an individual patient. This study highlights the dilemma of such practice, where patients deemed futile by predictive scores and physician opinion could still have meaningful recovery with aggressive medical therapy. Furthermore, the overestimation of these predictive scores, which can sway physician opinion, is likely due to inclusion of patients who had medical care withdrawn. The decision to withdraw care occurred early in hospitalization and was the strongest predictor of mortality. The study reinforces the importance of a case-by-case clinical approach.

Question

Should all patients with ICH and poor predictive scores have care withdrawn?

Answer

No, patients with poor ICH predictive scores can have meaningful neurologic recovery with maximal medical therapy.

rtPA FOR INTRAVENTRICULAR HEMORRHAGE

Low-Dose Recombinant Tissue-Type Plasminogen Activator Enhances Clot Resolution in Brain Hemorrhage

Naff N, Williams MA, Keyl PM, et al. *Stroke*. 2011;42(11):3009–3016

BACKGROUND

IVH occurs in up to 40% of ICH cases and is associated with higher mortality than ICH alone. Worse outcomes are due to ventricular blood products causing direct neurotoxicity, infections, and hydrocephalus necessitating placement of extraventricular drains (EVD) to avoid herniation. Despite reduction of intracranial pressure from EVDs, patients do not always improve, and it is not until blood products substantially resolve that mental status is more likely to recover. Animal models suggest faster clot resolution in IVH results in improved neurologic outcomes, which prompted observational studies, small clinical trials, and meta-analyses suggesting benefit with intraventricular clot lysis. Ultimately, RCTs were initiated to evaluate safety and efficacy of low-dose recombinant tissue–type plasminogen activator (rtPA) in IVH.

OBJECTIVES

To determine safety and efficacy of rtPA administered via EVD for the treatment of IVH.

METHODS

Randomized, prospective, open treatment, phase 2 trial involving 14 neurology intensive care units (ICUs) in the United States.

Patients

Forty-eight patients with ICH and massive IVH who already had EVD placement were randomized to receive intraventricular rtPA ($n = 26$) or saline placebo ($n = 22$). Inclusion criteria included 18 to 75 years of age, supratentorial ICH, and small ICH volume of <30 mL. Exclusion criteria included infratentorial or subtentorial ICH, pregnancy, tumor, coagulopathy, or vascular etiology of bleed. Patients received daily head CT imaging to assess for asymptomatic bleeding and clot resolution, with a follow-up CT at days 28 to 32. The intraventricular injections were continued every 12 hours or until clot resolution allowed removal of EVD or until safety end points were reached (i.e., bleeding, ventriculitis, or death).

Interventions

rtPA (3 mg/3 mL) vs. normal saline (3 mL) injected into ventricles through an extant EVD.

Outcomes

Primary outcomes were safety end points of mortality, ventriculitis, and bleeding. Secondary outcomes included rate of clot lysis with linear regression analysis modeling effect on GCS.

KEY RESULTS

- No significant difference in mortality, ventriculitis, or symptomatic bleeding between both cohorts. Of note, symptomatic bleeding was 23% in the treatment arm compared to 5% in placebo ($p = 0.10$).
- Significantly faster blood clot lysis in the rtPA arm compared to placebo (18% per day vs. 8% per day, $p < 0.001$).
- 10% per day increase in the rate of clot resolution was associated with a 1.1 point improvement in GCS 96 hours after the initial GCS (95% CI = 0.49–1.63, $p < 0.001$).
- No significant difference in average days of infusion of rtPA vs. placebo (10.2 and 12.7 days, respectively).

STUDY CONCLUSIONS

3 mg rtPA can be safely infused into EVDs for IVH with faster blood clot lysis but trend toward higher risk of bleeding with unclear long-term benefit.

COMMENTARY

Given the substantial mortality of IVH, efforts to improve outcomes have accelerated. This randomized study from 2011 established the safety of the rtPA while also demonstrating faster clot lysis with modeled effects on sooner GCS improvement. The CLEAR-IVH (part A and B) trials were published in 2008 establishing dosing safety profiles of rtPA. Although important for establishing safety, these trials did not illuminate if rtPA conferred any long-term benefit. Thus, the CLEAR III trial was initiated in 2008 to follow IVH patients receiving rtPA for up to 12 months to assess functional outcomes.

Question

Does rtPA provide short-term benefit for IVH over placebo?

Answer

No, although rtPA can be given safely, short-term benefit is not superior to placebo and long-term benefit remains unclear.

CHAPTER 30

GRADING OF RUPTURED SUBARACHNOID HEMORRHAGES

David J. Lin ∎ Steven M. Greenberg

Surgical Risk as Related to Time of Intervention in the Repair of Intracranial Aneurysms

Hunt WE, Hess RM. *Neurosurgery*. 1968;28(1):14–20

Relation of Cerebral Vasospasm to Subarachnoid Hemorrhage Visualized by Computerized Tomographic Scanning

Fisher CM, Kistler JP, Davis JM, et al. *Neurosurgery*. 1980;6(1):1–9

BACKGROUND

The optimal time to operate on and the surgical risk for patients with ruptured intracranial aneurysms with subarachnoid hemorrhage depend on a number of factors including the amount of subarachnoid blood, the patient's clinical condition at the time of surgery, and the location of the aneurysm. These two historic studies examined clinical and radiographic criteria for grading ruptured saccular aneurysms and subsequently correlated their grading scales with clinical outcome (delayed neurologic deterioration, vasospasm, and mortality).

OBJECTIVES

Hunt and Hess applied clinical criteria that included the (1) intensity of the meningeal inflammatory reaction, (2) the severity of the neurologic deficit, and (3) the presence or absence of significant associated disease to create a 5-point clinical grading scale in order to evaluate surgical risk and selection for patients with ruptured intracranial aneurysms. Fisher et al. investigated the relationship between the amount and distribution of subarachnoid blood detected by CT scan and the later development of cerebral vasospasm.

METHODS

	Hunt and Hess	Fisher, Kistler, and Davis
Patients:	Retrospective study of 275 patients treated at Ohio State University over a 12-year period	Retrospective study of 47 cases of aneurysmal rupture with CT scans performed within the first 5 days after subarachnoid hemorrhage

	Hunt and Hess	**Fisher, Kistler, and Davis**
Classification:	The 5-point clinical grading scale was as follows: (I) Asymptomatic, minimal headache, slight nuchal rigidity. (II) Moderate to severe headache, nuchal rigidity, no neurologic deficit other than cranial nerve palsy. (III) Drowsiness, confusion, or mild focal deficit. (IV) Stupor, moderate to severe hemiparesis, possible early decerebrate rigidity, and vegetative disturbances. (V) Deep coma, decerebrate rigidity, moribund appearance. Note that Grade I and II patients were taken to surgery as soon as diagnosis could be made. Grade III or below patients were treated conservatively until they improved to Grade I or II	Subarachnoid blood on CT scan was classified into four grades: (1) no blood detected, (2) a diffuse deposition of thin layers, with all vertical layers of bleed less than 1 mm thick, (3) localized clots and/or vertical layers of bleed 1 mm or greater in thickness, (4) diffuse or no subarachnoid blood, but with intracerebral or intraventricular blood
Outcomes:	The primary outcomes analyzed were operative and nonoperative mortality. Secondary outcomes included infarction and rebleeding rates	The primary outcome measures were the amount and severity of vasospasm. Clinical signs corresponding to vasospasm were also recorded
Key Results:	• Grade I and II patients had an overall mortality rate of 20% and an operative mortality rate of 14%. • The majority of nonoperative deaths were caused by rebleeding. • Grade II patients had a much higher mortality rate as compared to grade I patients (22% vs. 1.4%), and the major source of this increased mortality was cerebral infarction secondary to vasospasm. • 55% of Grade III patients (subjected to delayed surgical intervention) improved to Grade I or II after delaying surgical intervention. • The primary cause of mortality in Grade III patients was cerebral infarction.	• Vasospasm almost exclusively and invariably occurred in patients with globular clots (larger than 5 × 3 mm) or subarachnoid blood ≥1 mm thick in the fissures and vertical cisterns. • Conversely, patients without large subarachnoid blood clots and thick layers of blood did not experience vasospasm. • Almost all patients with severe vasospasm showed signs of ischemia in the cerebral territories corresponding to the vasospastic arteries.

STUDY CONCLUSIONS

Surgery for patients without significant clinical neurologic sequelae of subarachnoid hemorrhage from a ruptured intracranial aneurysm carries relatively low risk. Half of the patients with significant neurologic deficits (i.e., stupor, Grade III and above) will improve clinically and at this point may be better operative candidates. Patients at high risk for vasospasm can be clearly identified by the amount and location of subarachnoid blood on CT scan.

COMMENTARY

Subarachnoid hemorrhage from a ruptured intracranial aneurysm is a significant source of morbidity and mortality. The timing of surgery to secure a ruptured aneurysm after subarachnoid hemorrhage continues to be an important issue. Early aneurysm clipping prevents rebleeding, a major cause of death after subarachnoid hemorrhage. On the other hand, this needs to be balanced with the safety of early surgery, particularly with undetected vasospasm leading to cerebral ischemia. These two landmark retrospective studies provide a framework for clinically and radiographically grading patients with aneurysmal subarachnoid hemorrhage. Clinically, the Hunt and Hess study separates patients based on their neurologic examination into those who would likely benefit from early surgery (patients without significant neurologic sequelae from initial bleed) and those for whom surgery could be delayed to allow for improvement in their initially poor neurologic examination. Radiographically, Fisher et al. showed patients could be stratified into groups by subarachnoid blood volume as a proxy for increased vasospasm risk. Moreover, Fisher et al. demonstrated how location of subarachnoid blood predicts neurologic deficits after vasospasm. In practice today, most neurovascular surgeons operate within 3 to 4 days of aneurysmal bleeding in good grade patients to minimize rebleeding. The surgical practice with regard to poor grade patients (significantly neurologically affected) remains variable, and interventional methods for securing aneurysms early have further confounded practice.

Question

Can we use clinical and radiographic criteria to risk-stratify patients with subarachnoid hemorrhage from a ruptured intracranial aneurysm?

Answer

Yes, CT scan findings predict vasospasm and patients can, on a first pass, be risk stratified for surgery based on neurologic examination.

SECTION 3

TRAUMATIC BRAIN INJURY

Brian L. Edlow ■ Daniel B. Rubin

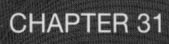

CHAPTER 31 | GLASGOW COMA SCALE

Assessment of Coma and Impaired Consciousness: A Practical Scale
Teasdale G, Jennett B. *Lancet.* 1974;304(7872):81–84

BACKGROUND
In traumatic brain injury (TBI) and other severe neurologic diseases, the level of consciousness is often the most significant clinical sign by which treatment and prognosis is guided. However, level of consciousness may be characterized using imprecise and subjective terminology, making it difficult to detect longitudinal changes in the neurologic examination or to reliably track patient outcomes. A simple clinical scale based on objective, easily reproducible exam findings was thus developed to aid in the assessment of consciousness after TBI.

OBJECTIVES
To develop a practical scoring system that can be used by both experts and nonexperts to rapidly and reproducibly characterize the level of consciousness in patients with brain injuries.

METHODS
Uncontrolled observational study of patients admitted to a tertiary care hospital in Scotland in 1974.

Patients
Patients admitted with decreased level of consciousness in the setting of brain injury.

Interventions
Patients were assessed on three axes of behavioral responses: eye opening, motor responses, and verbal responses. The initial GCS, as proposed in this chapter, is a 14-point scale (1 to 4 for eye opening, 1 to 5 for motor response, 1 to 5 for verbal response); however, the modern GCS (revised by the authors of this chapter in 1976) is a 15-point scale (included below).

	Eye Opening	Verbal Response	Motor Response
1	Does not open eyes	None	No response
2	Opens eyes to noxious stimuli	Incomprehensible speech	Extensor (decerebrate) posturing
3	Opens eyes to voice	Inappropriate speech	Flexor (decorticate) posturing
4	Spontaneously opens eyes	Confused and/or disoriented	Withdraws from painful stimulus
5		Appropriately conversant	Localizes to painful stimulus
6			Follows commands

Outcomes

The primary outcome was the reproducibility of the score assigned to each patient and agreement between examiners.

KEY RESULTS

- After having several doctors and nurses examine patients and assign each a score on the GCS, disagreements between examiners were "rare" (no interrater reliability data are provided).

STUDY CONCLUSIONS

The GCS may be useful as a tool for rapidly and reproducibly describing the level of consciousness in patients with brain injuries.

COMMENTARY

Although not a clinical trial, the original description of the GCS is included in this collection because it was the first attempt to quantify and rigorously characterize level of consciousness, and in doing so transformed the care of patients with head trauma and other severe brain injuries. Using the GCS, clinicians could more quickly and accurately communicate about a patient's neurologic status and make more objective decisions regarding the need for medical and surgical interventions. In addition, the GCS served as a powerful tool for future clinical investigations; indeed, virtually all of the other studies on TBI in this collection enrolled patients based on their admission GCS scores. One of the key points made by the authors is that this scale does not attempt to distinguish who is or is not conscious, but rather simply provides a way to describe the level of consciousness in a clear and reproducible manner.

Question

Can disorders of consciousness be described by both neurologists and nonspecialists using a quick, reproducible examination scale?

Answer

Yes, the GCS was designed specifically for that purpose.

CHAPTER 32

ALBUMIN VS. SALINE FOR RESUSCITATION AFTER TRAUMATIC BRAIN INJURY

Saline or Albumin for Fluid Resuscitation in Patients with Traumatic Brain Injury

The SAFE Study Investigators. *NEJM*. 2007;357(9):874–884

BACKGROUND

The SAFE trial (2004) investigated outcomes in intensive care unit (ICU) patients resuscitated with albumin vs. saline. Although no significant difference between the two groups was observed overall, a subgroup analysis suggested an increased mortality in TBI patients resuscitated with albumin. The present study was designed to investigate the difference in outcomes in TBI patients who were resuscitated with albumin vs. saline.

OBJECTIVES

To determine the difference in outcome for TBI patients who receive fluid resuscitation with albumin vs. saline.

METHODS

A post hoc analysis of a multicenter, double-blind, RCT conducted in 16 hospitals in Australia and New Zealand between 2001 and 2003.

Patients

460 patients, age 18 years and older, who were admitted with a GCS score of 13 or less, and an abnormality on head CT consistent with a diagnosis of TBI.

Interventions

Eligible patients were randomized to receive either 4% albumin or normal saline for all fluid resuscitation in the ICU until death, discharge, or 28 days from randomization.

Outcomes

The primary outcomes were mortality and functional neurologic outcome at 24 months after randomization, as measured by the Extended Glasgow Outcome Scale (GOSE). Favorable outcome was defined as a GOSE score of 5 to 8 and unfavorable outcome as a GOSE score of 1 to 4.

KEY RESULTS

- At 24 months, mortality in the albumin group was 33.2% and mortality in the saline group was 20.4% (relative risk = 1.63 [1.17–2.26], >85% of deaths occurred within the first 28 days).

- In the subgroup of patients with severe TBI (GCS = 3–8), mortality in the albumin vs. saline groups was 41.8% vs. 22.2% (relative risk = 1.88 [1.31–2.70]). There was no difference in mortality in patients with moderate TBI (GCS = 9–12).
- There were fewer favorable outcomes in the albumin group compared to the saline group (47.3% vs. 60.6%, relative risk = 0.78 [0.65–0.94]).

STUDY CONCLUSIONS
Higher mortality is observed among patients with severe TBI who receive fluid resuscitation with 4% albumin than among those who receive saline.

COMMENTARY

For decades the field of critical care medicine had been divided over whether colloid or crystalloid was the optimal fluid to administer for resuscitation in the ICU. Given albumin's higher oncotic load, less total volume is needed to replenish the intravascular compartment and achieve a target blood pressure. With less fluid entering the interstitial space, there is less third spacing and theoretically a decreased risk of pulmonary edema as well. However, hypovolemia not due to bleeding often involves a fairly significant loss of fluid from the interstitial space as well, which is more adequately resuscitated with saline. The original SAFE trial examined outcomes for fluid resuscitation with albumin vs. saline in a large heterogeneous population of ICU patients. The presently discussed study was designed to analyze the head trauma subpopulation of the SAFE trial in more detail, and follow outcomes out to 2 years. Consistent with the findings of the original SAFE trial, TBI patients treated with albumin did markedly worse than those treated with saline. The mechanism underlying this drastic difference in outcomes is still unknown, although it may be due to a coagulopathy induced by high doses of exogenous albumin. Importantly, because this study was a post hoc analysis, caution must be taken to prevent overinterpretation. Such a study can demonstrate an association between treatment arms and outcomes, but cannot, by definition, be used as evidence of a causal relationship.

Question
Does the type of fluid used for resuscitation in TBI influence outcome?

Answer
Yes, TBI patients resuscitated with 4% albumin have a significantly increased mortality rate compared to patients resuscitated with normal saline.

CHAPTER 33

DECOMPRESSIVE CRANIECTOMY IN TRAUMATIC BRAIN INJURY

Decompressive Craniectomy in Diffuse Traumatic Brain Injury

Cooper JD, Rosenfeld JV, Murray L, et al. *NEJM*. 2011;364(16):1493–1502

BACKGROUND
Decompressive craniectomy is often used to treat refractory intracranial hypertension in TBI. It is unknown whether this surgical intervention improves outcomes.

OBJECTIVES
To determine the effect of decompressive craniectomy on functional outcome in patients with TBI.

METHODS
Multicenter RCT conducted at 15 tertiary care hospitals in Australia, New Zealand, and Saudi Arabia between 2002 and 2010.

Patients
155 adults, age 15 to 59 years, admitted with severe nonpenetrating TBI (GCS score 3 to 8 after resuscitation/before intubation or Marshall class III on head CT) with intracranial hypertension (>20 mm Hg for 15 minutes in a 1-hour period) refractory to first-line treatments. Patients with spinal cord injuries, mass lesions requiring surgery, dilated and unreactive pupils, or cardiac arrest were excluded.

Interventions
Eligible patients were randomized within 72 hours after injury either to undergo bifrontotemporoparietal craniectomy with bilateral dural opening plus standard care or standard care alone. Standard care second-tier medical treatment for intracranial hypertension included mild hypothermia and barbiturates.

Outcomes
The primary outcomes were the proportion of patients with an unfavorable outcome (a score of 1 to 4 on the Extended Glasgow Outcome Scale [GOSE]) at 6 months and the absolute score on GOSE at 6 months. Secondary outcomes were intracranial pressure (ICP), the percentage of time with intracranial hypertension, the number of days in the ICU and hospital, the proportion of patients with severe disability (GOSE = 2 to 4) at 6 months, and mortality at 6 months.

KEY RESULTS

- Six months after injury, outcomes in the craniectomy group were worse than in the standard care group (median GOSE 3 vs. 4, odds ratio [OR] for a worse outcome 1.84 [1.05–3.24]).
- In the craniectomy group, unfavorable outcomes occurred in 70% of patients vs. 51% in the standard care group (OR = 2.21 [1.14–4.26]).
- After randomization, the mean ICP and amount of time with intracranial hypertension was lower in the craniectomy group compared to the standard care group (mean ICP was 14.4 ± 6.8 mm Hg vs. 19.1 ± 8.9 mm Hg, and the median number of hours with ICP > 20 mm Hg was 9.2 [IQR = 4.4–27.0] vs. 30.0 [IQR = 14.9–60.0]).

STUDY CONCLUSIONS

Despite having a significantly lower ICP, patients who underwent decompressive craniectomy for the treatment of intracranial hypertension refractory to first-line treatments had a worse outcome than patients who received standard care alone.

COMMENTARY

This trial was the first to examine the utility of decompressive craniectomy for the treatment of elevated ICP in TBI in a prospective, controlled manner. The results were surprising for two reasons: not only did patients who underwent craniectomy have worse outcomes, but these outcomes occurred despite a substantial improvement in ICP control. These findings suggest that perhaps ICP control alone is not sufficient in the management of TBI. Despite randomization, the two study groups in this trial differed significantly in the proportion of patients with unreactive pupils (with a greater proportion in the surgery arm), suggesting on average more severe baseline brainstem injuries. In a post hoc multivariate analysis that attempted to correct for this difference, the primary outcomes between the two groups were no longer significantly different. Additionally, a liberal definition of "refractory" intracranial hypertension may have confounded the duration of MM prior to considering surgical intervention. Such a low threshold may have led to the comparison of patients with a transient ICP rise to those consigned to an aggressive neurosurgical intervention. Additionally, the high morbidity rate of bifrontotemporoparietal craniectomy has been brought up as a potential contributor to the results and many neurosurgeons choose to perform a hemicraniectomy instead. Given these caveats, the impact of this trial on clinical practice has been mixed. Although bifrontotemporoparietal craniectomy is now less commonly performed, anecdotal evidence suggests that hemicraniectomy may be a life-saving intervention in severe TBI patients who have refractory intracranial hypertension.

Question

Does decompressive bifrontotemporoparietal craniectomy for refractory intracranial hypertension improve outcomes in severe TBI?

Answer

No, patients who undergo decompressive bifrontotemporoparietal craniectomy for refractory intracranial hypertension have worse outcomes than patients treated with standard medical therapy alone.

CHAPTER 34

ANTIEPILEPTIC DRUGS AFTER TRAUMATIC BRAIN INJURY

A Randomized, Double-Blind Study of Phenytoin for the Prevention of Post-Traumatic Seizures

Temkin NR, Dikmen SS, Wilensky AJ, et al. *NEJM*. 1990;323(8):497–502

BACKGROUND

Seizures are a major source of long-term morbidity after TBI. Earlier retrospective and randomized prospective trials offered mixed evidence on the effectiveness of phenytoin at reducing the long-term rates of posttraumatic seizures. This study was the first to prospectively investigate the efficacy of prophylactic phenytoin for the prevention of seizures after TBI.

OBJECTIVES

To determine the effectiveness of early treatment with phenytoin to prevent the occurrence of posttraumatic seizures.

METHODS

Randomized, double-blind, placebo-controlled trial conducted at an urban Level 1 trauma center between 1983 and 1987.

Patients

404 patients, age 16 or older, who presented within 24 hours of severe head injury defined as a cortical contusion visible on CT scan; a subdural, epidural, or intracerebral hematoma; a depressed skull fracture, a penetrating head wound, a seizure within 24 hours of injury, or a score of 10 or less on the GCS. Patients with a history of prior head trauma, seizures, "severe alcoholism" or prior neurologic condition that may predispose to seizures, or prior neurosurgery were excluded.

Interventions

Patients were randomized to receive either phenytoin or placebo in a double-blind fashion and followed clinically for 2 years. Patients randomized to the treatment arm received a loading dose of IV phenytoin followed by maintenance drug for 12 months. Serum phenytoin levels were monitored regularly and dose adjustments were made to maintain serum levels in the high therapeutic range.

Outcomes

The primary outcome was the occurrence of seizures, which were classified as either early (within 7 days of drug loading) or late (occurring after 7 days). Secondary outcomes were possible adverse drug effects of phenytoin.

KEY RESULTS

- Early treatment with prophylactic phenytoin led to a significant reduction in early seizure rates (3.6% vs. 14.2%, risk ratio = 0.27 [0.12–0.62]), but did not yield a significant reduction in the incidence of late seizures.
- At the end of the 2-year observation period, the incidence of seizures in the phenytoin and placebo group was 27.5% and 21.1%, respectively ($p > 0.2$).
- There was no difference in either early or late mortality between the treatment and placebo groups.

STUDY CONCLUSIONS

Phenytoin reduces the incidence of seizures in the first week after TBI, but does not reduce the incidence of seizures thereafter.

COMMENTARY

Prior to this study, patients were routinely discharged from the hospital on prolonged courses of antiepileptic drugs (AEDs) with the belief that they would prevent epileptogenesis. This trial was significant because it showed that although prophylactic AEDs were effective at reducing the rate of early posttraumatic seizures, they had no effect on late posttraumatic seizures. Following the publication of this trial, the routine practice of discharging trauma patients on long courses of AEDs was largely abandoned. Despite being a largely negative trial, this study did demonstrate a powerful and important effect of prophylactic AED therapy at reducing early seizures. Although they are not synonymous with posttraumatic epilepsy, early seizures can be intrinsically dangerous, as they can cause increased intracranial pressure and contribute to secondary injury. Thus, there is value in preventing these early, and it is now standard practice to treat all severe TBI patients prophylactically with a 7-day course of AEDs. Posttraumatic epileptogenesis remains an area of active research; since the publication of this study, other trials have explored the role of carbamazepine, magnesium sulfate, and corticosteroids in preventing post-TBI epilepsy. Unfortunately, these trials have all been negative as well.

Question

Does prophylactic treatment with phenytoin after head injury prevent the development of posttraumatic epilepsy?

Answer

No. There is no long-term difference in posttraumatic seizure incidence between patients treated with phenytoin and placebo.

CHAPTER 35

INTRACRANIAL PRESSURE MONITORING IN TRAUMATIC BRAIN INJURY

A Trial of Intracranial-Pressure Monitoring in Traumatic Brain Injury

Chesnut RM, Temkin N, Carney N, et al. *NEJM*. 2012;367(26):2471–2481

BACKGROUND

Invasive ICP monitoring is considered the standard of care for the management of severe TBI. However, the efficacy of invasive pressure monitoring to improve outcome has not been demonstrated in a controlled trial.

OBJECTIVES

To determine the efficacy of using invasive ICP monitoring to guide therapy in TBI.

METHODS

Randomized, prospective, parallel-group trial conducted at six South American hospitals between 2008 and 2012.

Patients

324 patients, age 13 years or older, who presented with a severe TBI defined as GCS score 3 to 8 (or GCS motor subscale 1 to 5 for intubated patients) or in whom GCS decreased into the eligibility range within 48 hours of presentation. Patients with injuries deemed unsurvivable or with GCS 3 and bilateral fixed and dilated pupils were excluded.

Interventions

Patients were randomized to either the "pressure-monitoring" group or the "imaging-clinical examination" group. Patients in the pressure-monitoring group had an intraparenchymal pressure monitor placed and were treated with a protocolized regimen of therapy for elevated ICP, including hyperosmolar therapy, sedation, mild hyperventilation, and external ventricular drain (EVD) placement for cerebrospinal fluid (CSF) diversion, with a goal ICP < 20 mm Hg. Patients in the imaging-clinical examination group received the same treatments, with decision-making guided by clinical examinations and CT scans in accordance with the pretrial standard of care at participating hospitals.

Outcomes

The primary outcome was a composite of survival time, duration and level of impaired consciousness, functional status at 3 and 6 months (as measured by the Extended Glasgow Outcome Scale (GOSE), the Disability Rating Scale, and the Galveston Orientation and Amnesia Test (GOAT)), and neuropsychologic status at 6 months. Secondary outcomes included length of ICU stay, duration and total amount of "brain-specific" therapy, and systemic complications.

KEY RESULTS

- At 6 months, there was no difference in the primary outcome between the two groups ($p = 0.49$).
- The 6-month mortality was 41% in the imaging-clinical examination group and 39% in the pressure-monitoring group ($p = 0.6$).
- There was no difference in the length of ICU stay between the two groups; however, patients in the imaging-clinical examination group did receive significantly more days of "brain-specific" therapy.

STUDY CONCLUSIONS

The use of ICP monitoring to guide therapy does not improve outcomes in TBI.

COMMENTARY

The 2007 guidelines of the Brain Trauma Foundation recommend the placement of an ICP monitor in any patient admitted with a severe TBI (GCS $\leq$ 8), who meets the following criteria: CT scan demonstrating hematomas, contusions, swelling, herniation, or compressed basal cisterns; age >40 years, unilateral or bilateral motor posturing, or systolic blood pressure <90 mmHg. Given the wide adoption of this practice in the United States, the trial was conducted in South America, where ICP monitors are neither routinely placed nor the standard of care. The results of this study must be interpreted in their unique clinical context, as differences in resources and medical infrastructure may confound the principal finding. In particular, the authors highlight that no patient had access to postdischarge rehabilitation. Additionally, this trial did not question the efficacy of treating elevated ICP; rather, it evaluated whether or not an invasive monitor was superior to the clinical exam and CT scan to assess for elevated ICP. The observation that patients with invasive monitors received less "brain-specific" therapy suggests that the absence of an ICP monitor leads to more aggressive treatment to achieve the same outcome. Although ICP monitors remain standard of care for severe TBI patients in the United States, this trial's results suggest that there may be equipoise between invasive and noninvasive management of increased ICP to conduct a siremoveumilar trial in the United States.

Question

Does the use of an invasive ICP monitor to guide treatment improve outcome in severe TBI?

Answer

No, the use of an ICP monitor to guide therapy may not improve outcome in TBI.

CHAPTER 36

AMANTADINE FOR RECOVERY OF CONSCIOUSNESS AFTER TRAUMATIC BRAIN INJURY

Placebo-Controlled Trial of Amantadine for Severe Traumatic Brain Injury

Giacino JT, Whyte J, Bagiella E, et al. *NEJM*. 2012;366(9):819–826

BACKGROUND

Amantadine is commonly prescribed to patients with a prolonged decreased level of consciousness (i.e., vegetative state or minimally conscious state) after TBI in an effort to promote neurologic recovery. Limited data existed prior to 2012 to support this practice.

OBJECTIVES

To determine the effect of amantadine on functional neurologic recovery after TBI in patients with decreased level of consciousness.

METHODS

Randomized, double-blind, placebo-controlled trial conducted at 11 clinical sites in three countries.

Patients

184 patients, age 16 to 65 years, in a vegetative or minimally conscious state following a TBI within the past 4 to 16 weeks. Exclusion criteria included prior neurologic injury predating the TBI, medical instability, more than one seizure in the prior month, and significant renal insufficiency.

Interventions

Eligible participants were randomized to receive either amantadine or placebo for 4 weeks. Patients randomized to the treatment arm were treated with amantadine 100 mg twice daily for 2 weeks. The dose was increased to a maximum of 200 mg at weeks 3 and 4 if there was a less than 2-point improvement from baseline on the Disability Rating Scale (DRS) score.

Outcomes

The primary outcome was the rate of recovery, quantified by the slope of the DRS score over the 4 weeks of treatment. The second outcome was the durability of the treatment effect, quantified by the change in the DRS score during the 2-week washout period between weeks 4 and 6. Prespecified subgroup analyses divided patients by initial severity (vegetative vs. minimally conscious state) and time between injury and enrollment (4 to 10 weeks vs. 10 to 16 weeks).

KEY RESULTS

- Patients in the amantadine group experienced a faster rate of neurologic recovery during the 4 weeks of treatment. This effect persisted when patients were subdivided by initial severity (vegetative vs. minimally conscious state) and time from injury to enrollment (4 to 10 weeks vs. 10 to 16 weeks).
- During the 2-week washout period, the rate of recovery was significantly slower in the amantadine group than in the treatment group, and at the 6-week trial endpoint, there was no difference in the total improvement on the DRS score between the treatment and placebo groups.

STUDY CONCLUSIONS

Treatment with amantadine for disorders of consciousness after TBI accelerates functional recovery.

COMMENTARY

TBI is a major cause of long-term cognitive dysfunction, and many patients suffer from prolonged disorders of consciousness, including vegetative and minimally conscious states. Stimulant medications, such as amantadine, modafinil, and methylphenidate, are routinely prescribed with the belief that they may improve or at least accelerate functional recovery. Prior to this study, however, the data supporting their use were limited. This study was the first RCT to demonstrate a clear benefit to amantadine in TBI recovery. Although the data from this trial demonstrate acceleration in recovery during the 4 weeks of treatment, the short duration of the trial remains one of its limitations. Recovery of consciousness is a process that is routinely assessed over the course of months to years, and this study does not address whether the use of amantadine improves long-term neurologic function. However, if accelerated recovery allows patients to transition from inpatient rehabilitation to home sooner, this is still a significant gain. Studies with a longer duration of treatment and follow-up will be necessary to determine if stimulant medications such as amantadine improve long-term cognitive outcomes in patients with traumatic disorders of consciousness.

Question

Does amantadine accelerate recovery of consciousness after TBI?

Answer

Yes, amantadine accelerates the rate of recovery after TBI.

CHAPTER 37

FUNCTIONAL IMAGING IN VEGETATIVE STATES

Willful Modulation of Brain Activity in Disorders of Consciousness

Monti MM, Vanhaudenhuyse A, Coleman MR, et al. *NEJM*. 2010;362(7):579–589

BACKGROUND

Disorders of consciousness following severe brain injuries are challenging to diagnose. Some patients thought to be in a chronic vegetative or minimally consciousness state may be capable of higher-level cognitive functions. Functional magnetic resonance imaging (fMRI) may be able to detect "covert" brain activity indicative of preserved consciousness in these patients.

OBJECTIVES

To demonstrate the ability of fMRI to detect volitional brain activity in patients with severe brain injuries whose bedside examination suggests a vegetative or minimally conscious state.

METHODS

Controlled study of convenience samples enrolled at two major referral centers in the UK and Belgium between 2005 and 2009.

Patients

16 healthy control subjects and 54 patients with severe brain injuries (TBI, hypoxic-ischemic brain injury, encephalitis, meningitis, and stroke) in clinically diagnosed vegetative (23 patients) and minimally conscious (31 patients) states were enrolled. Patients who demonstrated excessive spontaneous movements (deemed unable to tolerate an MRI scan) or with paramagnetic implants that contraindicated MRI were excluded.

Interventions

Study participants underwent fMRI scans during which they were instructed to perform a motor imagery task (i.e., imagine hitting a tennis ball) and a spatial imagery task (i.e., imagine navigating a familiar environment). Activation of the supplemental motor areas and parahippocampal gyri, respectively, was measured for each task using fMRI. During a subsequent communication task, all healthy control subjects and one patient were asked "yes/no" questions and instructed to answer by performing either the motor or spatial imagery tasks, with motor imagery signifying a "yes" response and spatial imagery signifying a "no" response.

Outcomes

The primary outcome was the ability to willfully modulate brain activity using motor and spatial imagery in the supplemental motor areas and parahippocampal gyri, respectively. The second primary outcome was the ability to correctly answer "yes/no" questions using motor and spatial imagery.

KEY RESULTS

- All 16 control subjects and 5/54 patients could willfully modulate their brain activity using motor and/or spatial imagery. In all five patients with volitional brain activity, motor imagery was associated with significantly greater activation in the supplemental motor areas than in the parahippocampal gyri. In 4/5 patients, spatial imagery was associated with significantly greater activation in the parahippocampal gyri than in the supplemental motor areas.
- All 16 controls and one of the patients who had reliable responses during the imagery tasks could answer "yes/no" questions using motor and spatial imagery to indicate affirmative and negative responses. The single patient answered five of six autobiographic questions correctly (the response to the sixth question was not incorrect, but could not be decoded).
- All five patients that had reliable responses during the imagery tasks had suffered traumatic brain injuries. None of the patients who had suffered hypoxic-ischemic brain injuries or other forms of brain injury demonstrated volitional brain activity.
- Four of the five patients who were able to generate responses had previously been diagnosed with vegetative state (including the patient that was able to produce reliable "yes/no" responses on the communication task), indicating a higher level of consciousness than had previously been assessed.

STUDY CONCLUSIONS

In some patients with chronic disorders of consciousness after TBI, fMRI may be able to detect evidence of preserved consciousness absent on bedside examination.

COMMENTARY

Distinct neural networks regulate arousal and awareness, such that patients with severe brain injuries may exist in a state of chronic wakefulness without awareness (i.e., a vegetative state). Recovery of awareness marks the transition from a vegetative state to a minimally conscious state, whereas functionally accurate communication and/or functional object use indicates emergence from the minimally conscious state. As patients recover awareness along this spectrum of disorders of consciousness, their increased capacity for cognition may evade detection by bedside examination because of motor deficits that prevent self-expression. For these patients, the dissociation between cognition and motor function has been referred to as "covert cognition," or, more recently, "cognitive motor dissociation." In this study, the authors provide proof of principle that in a small subset of patients with chronic disorders of consciousness, fMRI may reveal volitional brain activity that was undetectable by clinical exam, suggesting cognitive motor dissociation. This study was also significant in showing that patients with severe TBI may be more likely to have cognitive motor dissociation, as evidenced by fMRI evidence of volitional brain activity. Ongoing fMRI research continues to explore the ways in which we can augment current clinical tools to more precisely diagnose and prognosticate for patients with chronic disorders of consciousness after severe brain injuries.

Question

Can imaging demonstrate evidence of awareness in patients with chronic disorders of consciousness after TBI?

Answer

Yes, fMRI can be used to demonstrate patterns of brain activation suggesting awareness in patients whose clinical exam suggests chronic vegetative or minimally conscious state.

CHAPTER 38

CORTICOSTEROIDS FOR TRAUMATIC BRAIN INJURY

Effect of Intravenous Corticosteroids on Death within 14 Days in 10008 Adults with Clinically Significant Head Injury (MRC CRASH Trial): Randomised Placebo-Controlled Trial

CRASH Trial Collaborators. *Lancet*. 2004;364(9442):1321–1328

BACKGROUND

Corticosteroids had been used for decades in the management of acute head injury to reduce the secondary effects of posttraumatic inflammation on the brain. Despite limited but promising data from acute spinal cord injury studies, prior to this trial, there existed no large, randomized clinical trial investigating the utility of corticosteroids in acute head injury.

OBJECTIVES

To determine the effect of IV corticosteroids on death and disability in acute head injury.

METHODS

Randomized, double-blind, placebo-controlled trial conducted by an international consortium of over 200 hospitals in 49 countries between 1999 and 2004.

Patients

10,008 patients, age 16 years or older, who presented within 8 hours of a clinically significant head injury, defined as a GCS score of 14 or less. Patients with a clear clinical indication or contraindication for corticosteroids were not randomized.

Interventions

Eligible patients were randomized to receive a 48-hour IV infusion of MP or placebo. Patients in the treatment arm received a 2 gram loading dose of MP over the first hour followed by 0.4 grams/hour for 48 hours.

Outcomes

The primary outcomes were death within 2 weeks of injury and death or disability at 6 months. Disability was defined using the Glasgow outcome scale. Prespecified subgroup analyses included subdividing primary outcomes based on time from injury to randomization (<1 h, 1–3 h, 3–8 h) and severity of injury based on GCS (severe 3–8, moderate 9–12, mild 13–14).

KEY RESULTS
- Within 2 weeks of randomization, 21% of the patients randomized to the corticosteroid group died, compared to 18% of the patients randomized to placebo (relative risk 1.18 [1.09–1.27]).
- The increased relative risk of death with corticosteroid treatment did not differ by injury severity (p = 0.22) or time from injury to randomization (p = 0.05).
- This trial was stopped early by the study's data monitoring committee because of a statistically significant increase in mortality in the treatment arm. Thus, 6-month death and disability data were not reported.

STUDY CONCLUSIONS
Corticosteroids do not confer a mortality benefit and should not be routinely used in the treatment of TBI.

COMMENTARY

Prior to the publication of this study, corticosteroids were routinely used in the management of TBI. The mechanistic basis for such treatment was compelling; though the damage from the initial injury may be irreversible, it is believed that much of the long-term neurologic damage after TBI comes from secondary injuries arising from inflammation and other intrinsic cellular processes. Following the publication of this study, however, there was a rapid change in the management of TBI, with an abandonment of empiric corticosteroids. The cause of increased mortality in the corticosteroid group remains uncertain. Potential explanations include the possibility of clinically significant hyperglycemia in the corticosteroid group or secondary adrenal insufficiency following the administration of extremely high dose of corticosteroid (21.2 grams of MP over 2 days) used in the treatment arm. Despite these findings, the search for secondary injury prevention continues, with more recent studies investigating the use of magnesium, erythropoietin, therapeutic hypothermia, and progesterone. Unfortunately, none of these interventions has been shown to be effective in improving outcomes after TBI.

Question
Should patients with TBI be treated prophylactically with corticosteroids?

Answer
No, patients who receive corticosteroids after head injury have a significantly increased mortality at 2 weeks.

CHAPTER 39

CORTICOSTEROIDS IN ACUTE SPINAL CORD INJURY

A Randomized, Controlled Trial of Methylprednisolone or Naloxone in the Treatment of Acute Spinal-cord Injury: Results of the Second National Acute Spinal Cord Injury Study

Bracken MB, Shepard MJ, Collins WF, et al. *NEJM*. 1990;322:1405–1411

Administration of Methylprednisolone for 24 or 48 Hours or Tirilazad Mesylate for 48 Hours in the Treatment of Acute Spinal Cord Injury: Results of the Third National Acute Spinal Cord Injury Randomized Controlled Trial

Bracken MB, Shepard MJ, Holford TR, et al. *JAMA*. 1997;277(20):1597–1604

Pharmacological Therapy of Spinal Cord Injury during the Acute Phase

Pointillart V, Petitjean ME, Wiart L, et al. *Spinal Cord*. 2000;38:71–76

BACKGROUND

Acute spinal cord injury often results in severe neurologic deficits. After the initial injury, a cascade of pathologic processes occurring over the first hours to days is believed to ultimately determine the extent of permanent disability. A number of experimental studies in animals have suggested that early pharmacologic intervention during this critical period may improve the potential for recovery; however, prospective data in humans are limited.

OBJECTIVES

All three trials were designed to determine the efficacy of IV methylprednisolone (MP) and other pharmacologic interventions to improve neurologic recovery after acute traumatic spinal cord injury.

METHODS

	Bracken et al.[1]	Bracken et al.[2]	Pointillart et al.[3]
Methods:	Randomized, double-blind placebo-controlled trial conducted at 10 trauma centers in the United States. Dates not given	Randomized, double-blind clinical trial conducted at 16 spinal cord injury centers in North America between 1991 and 1995	Randomized, double-blind placebo-controlled trial conducted in France between 1990 and 1995

	Bracken et al.[1]	Bracken et al.[2]	Pointillart et al.[3]
Patients:	487 patients age 13 years or older presenting within 12 hours of acute spinal cord injury. Patients with nerve root injury or cauda equina syndrome only, gunshot wounds, life-threatening injuries, opioid addiction, chronic corticosteroid therapy, and those treated with MP or naloxone prior to arrival were excluded	499 patients age 14 years or older presenting within 6 hours of acute spinal cord injury. Patients with depressed level of consciousness, medical contraindications, and prior spinal cord injury were excluded	106 patients age 15–65 years admitted within 8 hours of acute spinal cord injury. Patients with GCS < 13, hemodynamic instability, mean arterial pressure (MAP) < 60, nerve root injury or cauda equina syndrome only, or other medical contraindications were excluded
Interventions:	Patients were randomized to receive a bolus dose and 24-hour infusion of IV MP, a bolus dose and 24-hour infusion of IV naloxone, or placebo	All patients received a bolus dose of IV MP, and were then randomized to receive either a 24- or 48-hour infusion of IV MP or a 48-hour infusion of tirilazad mesylate	Patients were randomized to receive a bolus dose and 24-hour infusion of IV MP, a bolus dose and 24-hour infusion of IV nimodipine, IV MP and nimodipine, or placebo
Outcomes:	The primary outcome was improvement in neurologic function at 6 weeks and 6 months. Additional outcomes included other morbidities and mortality	The primary outcomes were improvement in motor function on neurologic exam at 6 weeks and 6 months and improvement in the Functional Independence Measure (FIM) at 6 weeks and 6 months	The primary outcome was improvement in neurologic function at 1 year measured on the ASIA motor, pinprick sensation, and pain scores. Additional outcomes included medical complications, duration of ICU stay, and duration of mechanical ventilation
Key Results:	• Patients that received IV MP within 8 hours of injury had a significant improvement in neurologic function at 6 weeks and 6 months compared to placebo. • There was no difference observed in neurologic outcome in patients treated with IV naloxone, placebo, or IV MP at >8 hours from the time of injury. • There was no difference in mortality or major morbidities between the three groups.	• In patients treated between 3 and 8 hours from the time of injury, those who received a 48-hour infusion of IV MP had significantly greater improvement in motor function than those treated with 24 hours of IV MP or 48 hours of tirilazad mesylate. • When treatment was started within 3 hours, there was no difference in improvement between the three groups. • Patients treated with 48 hours of IV MP had significantly higher rates of severe sepsis and pneumonia. • Mortality was similar between all groups.	• No difference in neurologic outcome was found between patients treated with IV MP, IV nimodipine, MP and nimodipine, or placebo. • Patients treated with IV MP had significantly higher rates of hyperglycemia.

(continued)

	Bracken et al.[1]	Bracken et al.[2]	Pointillart et al.[3]
Study Conclusions:	When given within 8 hours of injury, IV MP improves long-term neurologic outcome after acute spinal cord injury	When treatment is started at 3–8 hours from the time of injury, patients treated with 48 hours of IV MP have significant improvement in neurologic outcome when compared to patients treated for 24 hours or with tirilazad mesylate	Neither IV MP nor nimodipine improves outcome after acute spinal cord injury

COMMENTARY

Acute spinal cord injury is a devastating condition that can cause permanent neurologic dysfunction. Despite impressive improvements in postinjury rehabilitation, there is still no definitive treatment to reliably improve neurologic function. Animal experiments from the 1960s and 1970s demonstrated enhanced recovery from spinal cord injury after treatment with corticosteroids. These findings led to the routine practice of treating patients with spinal cord injury with steroids. However, prior to the NASCIS II trial,[1] there were no high-quality data demonstrating the efficacy of such treatment in humans. Although the NASCIS II trial was technically a positive trial, many of the improvements noted were marginal, and many of the "positive" findings of the study failed to reach statistical significance. Additionally, this paper did not report the rates of surgical intervention between groups, which may have had a significant influence on outcome. Nonetheless, following the publication of this trial, treatment with high-dose IV MP quickly became the standard of care for acute spinal cord injury. The NASCIS III[2] trial expanded upon this work, demonstrating improved outcome with a longer course of IV MP in selected patients. Given the modest findings in both of these trials, however, skepticism regarding the efficacy of IV MP persisted. As the third of the trials discussed here[3] demonstrates, the data are mixed, and the best treatment for these patients is at present unknown. Importantly, a large and influential study conducted since the publication of these trials demonstrated a significantly increased mortality in TBI patients treated with corticosteroids (see the summary of the MRC CRASH trial). Because many patients with spinal cord injury also suffer from TBI, the use of corticosteroids in spinal cord injury has dwindled and is now not routinely recommended.

Question

Are there any pharmacologic treatments that definitively improve neurologic outcome after acute spinal cord injury?

Answer

No, at present no treatment has been shown to definitively improve neurologic recovery after acute spinal cord injury.

References

1. Bracken MB, Shepard MJ, Collins WF, et al. A randomized, controlled trial of methylprednisolone or naloxone in the treatment of acute spinal-cord injury: results of the second national acute spinal cord injury study. *NEJM*. 1990;322:1405–1411.
2. Bracken MB, Shepard MJ, Holford TR, et al. Administration of methylprednisolone for 24 or 48 hours or tirilazad mesylate for 48 hours in the treatment of acute spinal cord injury: results of the third national acute spinal cord injury randomized controlled trial. *JAMA*. 1997;277(20):1597–1604.
3. Pointillart V, Petitjean ME, Wiart L, et al. Pharmacological therapy of spinal cord injury during the acute phase. *Spinal Cord*. 2000;38:71–76.

Henrikas Vaitkevicius ■ David J. Lin

CHAPTER 40

MIDLINE SHIFT AND LEVEL OF CONSCIOUSNESS

Lateral Displacement of the Brain and Level of Consciousness in Patients with an Acute Hemispherical Mass

Ropper AH. *NEJM*. 1986;314:953–958

BACKGROUND

A central tenet of clinical neurology was that cerebral masses lead to alterations in consciousness by causing herniation of brain tissue. Uncal or central herniation syndromes causing compression of the reticular activating system or bihemispheric dysfunction, respectively, were believed to be the immediate cause of drowsiness, stupor, or coma. Modern-day CT scans allow for the opportunity to reassess these assumptions by correlating tissue shifts on imaging to clinical examination.

OBJECTIVES

To study brain-tissue shifts associated with alterations in consciousness in patients with acute unilateral cerebral masses using CT scan.

METHODS

Prospective observational cohort study of 24 patients admitted to the neurologic ICU with an acute supratentorial mass between July 1984 and August 1985.

Patients

Patients examined within 3 days of appearance of the mass were included in order to avoid the known tolerance of the brain to slowly enlarging masses. Causes of diminished alertness other than secondary tissue shifts were excluded. Patients who were initially comatose with fixed pupils were excluded.

Interventions

Patients were classified as awake, drowsy, stuporous, or comatose by clinical exam. CT scans were performed within 4 hours of the clinical examination, to detect the earliest radiographic changes.

Outcomes

Horizontal displacements of the center of the pineal body, cerebral aqueduct, and septum pellucidum were measured with a ruler on CT scans. Patency and widening of the cisterns surrounding the lower midbrain at the tentorial opening were considered evidence against transtentorial herniation.

KEY RESULTS

- Early depression of the level of alertness corresponded to distortion of the brain by horizontal displacement rather than transtentorial herniation.
- Horizontal displacement of the pineal body of 0 to 3 mm from the midline was associated with alertness, 3 to 4 mm with drowsiness, 6 to 8.5 mm with stupor, and 8 to 13 mm with coma.
- Drowsy or stuporous patients and some comatose patients had widened cisterns between the transtentorial edge and the midbrain on the side of the mass, suggesting that this space was not filled by herniated medial temporal lobe.
- Compression of one hemisphere by the other anteriorly (transfalcine herniation) was inconsistently related to alertness.

STUDY CONCLUSIONS

Alterations in consciousness with acute unilateral supratentorial masses were related to horizontal displacement rather than transtentorial herniation with brainstem compression. Current concepts of the anatomic and pathologic nature of depressed consciousness may require revision because they do not reflect early brain-tissue distortions.

COMMENTARY

This study examined the pathoanatomic relationship between alterations in level of consciousness and herniation syndromes. Traditionally, clinicians have been taught that stupor and coma are likely related to transtentorial or transfalcine herniation with resulting compression of the upper brainstem. This observational cohort study correlated CT findings with clinical exam in 24 patients with acute, unilateral cerebral masses and found that horizontal displacement, specifically of the pineal gland, rather than transtentorial herniation was strongly associated with depression of level of alertness (stupor and coma). The main limitations of the study were its small sample size, observational nature, and the human error associated with measuring lateral displacement of different brain structures. However, given the study objectives and its well-designed nature, the main conclusions are well worth considering. This study has helped clinicians to use CT scan findings to attribute decreased levels of consciousness in patients with an acute unilateral mass to either the mass itself, or search for alternative underlying causes of altered mental status.

Question

What is the underlying pathoanatomy of changes in levels of consciousness in patients with an acute hemispheral mass?

Answer

Horizontal lateral displacement rather than transtentorial herniation corresponds to stupor and coma in patients with acute unilateral cerebral masses.

CHAPTER 41

USE OF HYPEROSMOLAR THERAPY FOR CEREBRAL EDEMA

Management of Raised Intracranial Pressure and Hyperosmolar Therapy

Ropper AH. *NEJM*. 2014;14:152–158

BACKGROUND

Increased ICP is the final common pathway of many acute brain diseases including mass lesions, TBI, and ischemic or hemorrhagic strokes with cerebral edema and mass effect. Elevated ICP has consistently been associated with poor neurologic outcome and death. Because the cranium is a fixed vault, expansion of one of the intracranial components comes at the expense of reduction in other components (the Monro–Kellie hypothesis)—as brain volume increases, CSF is forced into the spinal subarachnoid spaces and cerebral blood flow is reduced. If unchecked, this process leads to global brain ischemia and brain death. Cerebral perfusion is defined as the mean arterial pressure (MAP) minus the sum of the ICP and venous pressure. The brain parenchyma is 80% water, making the brain very responsive to changes in water content. Hyperosmolar substances, with solutes that are excluded by the blood–brain barrier, reduce ICP by creating a gradient for water extraction from the brain.

OBJECTIVES

This review summarizes a series of landmark, historical studies describing the physiologic effects of and clinical experiences with specific chemical agents used with the goal of lowering ICP.

METHODS

Patients
NA

Interventions
NA

Outcomes
NA

KEY RESULTS
- Magnesium sulfate by mouth or by rectum is effective in decreasing ICP and thus controlling symptoms and signs of increased ICP.
- IV hypertonic sodium chloride solution was found to be effective for decreasing ICP during craniotomies.
- IV urea effectively reduced intracranial hypertension temporarily, but the effect of repeated administrations of urea remained in question.

- Mannitol may be effective in the following situations: (1) perioperatively to decrease intracranial tension when the dura mater is to be exposed, (2) temporary reversal of decompensating increased ICP and herniation, (3) cerebral edema after brain injury, and (4) pseudotumor cerebri.
- Oral administration of glycerol caused a rapid rise of plasma osmolality, an increase in diuresis, and a transient decrease in CSF pressure.
- Oral glycerol has been used postoperatively, in patients with head injury, and in patients with pseudotumor.
- 3% saline administration significantly lowered ICP 2 hours into infusion, whereas 0.9% saline administration did not in a pediatric TBI population.

STUDY CONCLUSIONS

Historically and still today, the mainstay of therapy for ICP remains focused on decreasing the water content of the brain by dehydration with hyperosmolar agents. The ideal osmotic agent and method of administration have not been established.

COMMENTARY
The administration of hyperosmolar agents for the reduction of elevated ICP has been explored since the 1920s. In clinical practice today, the two main agents most often used are mannitol and hypertonic saline based largely on the concepts demonstrated by these landmark studies (Table 41.1).[1-5] Mannitol is a sugar alcohol that causes sustained hyperosmolarity by diuresis and resulting dehydration, whereas hypertonic saline increases serum osmolarity directly. The ideal osmotic agent and method or interval of administration has not been established to date. Instead, the choice of hyperosmolar therapy is made practically based on blood pressure, cardiac output, and renal function, which guide the decision between a dehydrating osmotic agent (mannitol) and a volume-expanding salt solution (hypertonic saline). However, there is no evidence that there is a benefit to monitoring ICP as a means of directing hyperosmolar treatment and only sparse evidence that reducing ICP improves clinical outcomes.

Table 41.1 Summary of Historical Studies Evaluating Use of Hyperosmolar Therapies for Cerebral Edema

Faye[1]	Retrospective description and discussion of 16 patients who were given *magnesium sulfate* by mouth or rectum for signs of increased ICP as well as 15 patients who received a hypertonic salt solution intravenously to reduce ICP during neurosurgery for tumor resection.
Javid[2]	Described experience with and measured changes in CSF pressure in 21 patients who received *IV urea* for increased ICP.

(continued)

Table 41.1 Summary of Historical Studies Evaluating Use of Hyperosmolar Therapies for Cerebral Edema (*continued*)

Wise[3]	Described experience with patients who were given *hypertonic mannitol* solution to reduce ICP.
Buckell[4]	Reported on the physiologic effects of *glycerol* in normal human subjects and describes its clinical application in the treatment of patients with increased ICP.
Fisher[5]	18 pediatric patients with TBI were randomized to receiving *3% saline* vs. 0.9% saline for raised ICP. Outcome measures included ICP measured within 2 hours after administration, central venous pressure, renal function, and serum sodium concentration.

Question

Does hyperosmolar therapy reduce ICP?

Answer

Yes, but the optimal agent and dosing regimen, and whether there is a clear improvement in clinical outcomes, have yet to be definitively established.

References

1. Faye T. The administration of hypertonic salt solutions for the relief of intracranial pressure. *JAMA.* 1923;80(20):1445–1448.
2. Javid M, Settlage P. Effect of urea on cerebrospinal fluid pressure in human subjects. *JAMA.* 1956;160(11):943–949.
3. Wise B, Chater M. The value of hypertonic mannitol solution in decreasing brain mass and lowering cerebrospinal-fluid pressure. *J Neurosurg.* 1962;19(12):1038–1043.
4. Buckell M, Walsh L. Effects of glycerol by mouth on raised intracranial pressure in man. *Lancet.* 1964;2(7370):1151–1152.
5. Fisher B, Thomas D, Peterson B. Hypertonic saline lowers raised intracranial pressure in children after head trauma. *J Neurosurg Anesthesiol.* 1992;4(1):4–10.

CHAPTER 42

HYPERVENTILATION FOR ACUTE INTRACRANIAL PRESSURE ELEVATION

Changes in Human Cerebral Blood Flow Consequent on Alterations in Blood Gasses

Gibbs FA, Gibbs, EL, Lennox WG. *Am J Physiol*. 1935;111:557–563

BACKGROUND

Cerebral blood flow and autoregulation is a critical component of intracranial pressure. Prior to this historic paper, methods for measuring cerebral blood flow were limited and indirect. As a result, the mechanisms of changes in cerebral blood flow were largely unknown. Gibbs and colleagues used a thermoelectric blood flow recorder to measure the effect of changes in blood gas concentrations on cerebral blood flow.

OBJECTIVES

To report the effect of changes in the composition of respired air on cerebral blood flow in humans.

METHODS

A thermoelectric blood flow recorder inserted into the internal jugular vein was used to assess changes in blood flow in response to changes in blood gas concentrations.

Patients

Subjects were hospitalized patients who were not anesthetized. No further details of number of patients included or inclusion/exclusion criteria were given.

Interventions

Patients included in the study had thermoelectric blood flow recorders inserted into their internal jugular vein. The tip of the device was heated by an electric current to a temperature slightly higher than blood. The principle of the device was that if blood flowed faster past the tip, the tip would become cooler and, conversely, if blood slowed down, the tip would warm. The patients subsequently underwent hyperventilation (decreased CO_2), respiration of a gas mixture with 90% O_2 and 10% CO_2 (increased CO_2 content), respiration of nitrogen (decreased O_2 by proxy), or respiration of oxygen (increased O_2). There was no control group included.

Outcomes

Real-time changes in cerebral blood flow in response to changes in blood gas concentrations as measured by the thermoelectric blood flow recorded was the primary outcome. Changes in blood pressure were also measured.

KEY RESULTS

- Blowing off CO_2 by hyperventilation caused a decrease in cerebral blood flow.
- Breathing a high concentration of CO_2 resulted in an increase in cerebral blood flow.
- Anoxemia caused a distinct, but small increase in cerebral blood flow compared to effects of CO_2.
- There was no significant alteration in blood flow with respiration of pure oxygen.
- The observed changes in systemic arterial blood pressure were not significant in any case to account for changes in cerebral blood flow.

STUDY CONCLUSIONS

This observational study measured changes in cerebral blood flow in response to changes in carbon dioxide and oxygen tension using a thermoelectric blood flow recorder inserted in the internal jugular vein of unanesthetized human subjects. Increases in CO_2 increased cerebral blood flow, whereas decreases in CO_2 decreased cerebral blood flow, and systemic arterial blood pressure remained relatively constant. The authors hypothesize that the effects of CO_2 on cerebral blood flow are due to changes in the dilation of the cerebral vascular bed.

COMMENTARY

This historic study was made possible by the innovation of a thermoelectric blood flow recorder, which allowed real-time assessment of the effects of changes in blood gas concentration on cerebral blood flow. It laid the physiologic groundwork for future studies (i.e., by Nils Lundberg and others) that showed a reduction in ICP using hyperventilation. Over the years, the induction of respiratory alkalosis by hyperventilation has become a rapid and physiologically principled method for decreasing ICP in the acute setting. However, the effects of hyperventilation on cerebral blood flow are transient and, in the long term, outweighed by ischemic effects of cerebrovascular constriction. In addition, impaired cerebrovascular reactivity in neurocritical care populations, for example, TBI patients, limits the direct application of these physiologic principles.

Question

Do changes in carbon dioxide concentration affect cerebral blood flow?

Answer

Yes. Decreases in CO_2 induced by hyperventilation lead to decreased cerebral blood flow, and conversely increases in CO_2 lead to increased cerebral blood flow.

CHAPTER 43

TEMPERATURE MANAGEMENT FOR CARDIAC ARREST IN ADULTS

Mild Therapeutic Hypothermia to Improve the Neurologic Outcome after Cardiac Arrest

The Hypothermia after Cardiac Arrest Study Group. *NEJM*. 2002;346(8):549–556

Treatment of Comatose Survivors of Out-of-Hospital Cardiac Arrest with Induced Hypothermia

Bernard SA, Gray TW, Bust MD et al. *NEJM*. 2002;346(8):557–563

Targeted Temperature Management at 33°C versus 36°C after Cardiac Arrest

Nielsen N, Wetterslev J, Cronberg T, et al. *NEJM*. 2013;369(23):2197–2206

BACKGROUND

Cardiac arrest outside the hospital is common and has a poor prognosis. Unconscious survivors of out-of-hospital cardiac arrest often suffer from poor neurologic outcome. Therapeutic hypothermia, during which body temperature is lowered to a target level for a period of 24 hours, may preserve cerebral function and thus improve outcomes. Over the past decade, there have been three major RCTs studying whether hypothermia vs. normothermia and, subsequently, targeted temperature management at 33°C vs. 36°C improve neurologic outcome.

OBJECTIVES

The goal of the first two studies (both published in 2002) was to compare the effects of hypothermia to normothermia in unconscious patients after resuscitation from out-of-hospital cardiac arrest. The goal of the 2013 study was to compare hypothermia to 33°C vs. strict euthermia at 36°C.

METHODS

All three studies were multicenter randomized controlled studies.

	Mild Therapeutic Hypothermia to Improve the Neurologic Outcome after Cardiac Arrest	Treatment of Comatose Survivors of Out-of-Hospital Cardiac Arrest with Induced Hypothermia	Targeted Temperature Management at 33°C vs. 36°C after Cardiac Arrest
Patients:	Patients had to have witnessed ventricular fibrillation (VFib) or non-perfusing ventricular tachycardia cardiac arrest and an interval of <60 minutes from collapse to return of spontaneous circulation (ROSC). Major exclusion criteria were if patients were comatose before cardiac arrest or responded to verbal commands after ROSC	Patients had to have an initial rhythm of VFib and persistent coma after ROSC. Notable exclusion criteria were cardiogenic shock or possible causes of coma other than cardiac arrest	Patients with cardiac arrest irrespective of initial rhythm who were unconscious on admission were included. Main exclusion criteria were ROSC after >240 minutes, unwitnessed arrest with asystole, intracranial hemorrhage or stroke, and body temperature <30°C on admission
Interventions:	Patients were randomized to therapeutic hypothermia (core temperature between 32°C and 34°C) or to normothermia	Patients were randomized to hypothermia (core temperature to 33°C) or normothermia	Patients were randomized to a target body temperature of either 33°C or 36°C
Outcomes:	Primary outcome was favorable neurologic outcome (as measured by Pittsburgh cerebral-performance category) within 6 months after cardiac arrest. Secondary outcomes were morality within 6 months and rate of complications within 7 days	Primary outcome was survival to hospital discharge with sufficient neurologic function to be discharged home or to a rehabilitation facility. Secondary outcomes included the hemodynamic, biochemical, and hematologic effects of hypothermia	Primary outcome was all-cause mortality through the end of the trial. Secondary outcomes included poor neurologic function (as measured by cerebral performance category or modified Rankin scale) or death at 180 days
Key Results:	• 55% of patients in the hypothermia group vs. 39% in the normothermia group had favorable neurologic outcome (risk ratio, 1.40; 95% confidence interval, 1.08 to 1.81). • Mortality at 6 months was 41% in the hypothermia group as compared with 55% in the normothermia group (risk ratio 0.74; 95% confidence interval, 0.58 to 0.95). • The complication rate did not differ between the two groups.	• 49% of patients treated with hypothermia survived and had good outcome as compared with 26% of patients treated with normothermia ($p = 0.046$). • The OR for a good outcome with hypothermia as compared with normothermia was 5.25 (95% confidence interval 1.47 to 18.76). • There was no difference in the frequency of adverse events in the two groups.	• At the end of the trial, 50% of the patients in the 33°C group died as compared with 48% of the patients in the 36°C group ($p = 0.51$). • At 180-day follow-up, 54% of patients in the 33°C group had died or had poor neurologic function as compared to 52% of the patients in the 36°C group.

STUDY CONCLUSIONS

In patients who have been successfully resuscitated after cardiac arrest because of ventricular fibrillation, therapeutic hypothermia increased the rate of favorable neurologic outcome and reduced mortality. Treatment with moderate hypothermia appears to improve outcomes in patients with coma after resuscitation from out-of-hospital cardiac arrest. Hypothermia at a targeted temperature of 33°C did not confer a benefit as compared with strict euthermia at 36°C in unconscious survivors of out-of-hospital cardiac arrest.

COMMENTARY

Neurologic outcomes after cardiac arrest have traditionally been poor. This series of three landmark studies, all RCTs, showed significant benefit of hypothermia in terms of mortality and neurologic outcome. These findings have led to the widespread adoption of therapeutic hypothermia after cardiac arrest. Although the primary population studied in all three trials were out-of-hospital, ventricular fibrillation cardiac arrest patients, the practice has been extrapolated to often recommending hypothermia for other cardiac arrest populations (in-hospital cardiac arrest, initial rhythms other than VFib). Active cooling appears to be beneficial, but specific target temperatures seem less relevant as patients targeted to temperatures of 36°C did just as well as those cooled to 33°C. Additionally, the complications resulting from hypothermia itself such as shivering, increased sedation requirements, and medical complications (such as increased risk of bleeding and hypotension) must also be considered in the care of such patients. The optimal target temperature, timing, and duration of cooling have yet to be defined, and are subjects of active investigation. Furthermore, prognostication after cardiac arrest has become a much more complex topic in the era of therapeutic hypothermia.

Question

Does therapeutic hypothermia after cardiac arrest improve outcomes?

Answer

Yes. Therapeutic hypothermia after cardiac arrest improves neurologic outcome and reduces mortality.

CHAPTER 44

EARLY MOBILIZATION IN THE INTENSIVE CARE UNIT

Early Physical and Occupational Therapy in Mechanically Ventilated, Critically Ill Patients: A Randomized Controlled Trial

Schweickert WD, Pohlman MC, Pohlman AS, et al. *Lancet*. 2009;373(9678):1874–1882

BACKGROUND

Prolonged immobilization secondary to sedation significantly contributes to long-term complications of critical illness. Previous observational and cohort studies had suggested that early mobilization and minimization of sedation in the ICU shortens length of stay and decreases ICU-associated delirium.

OBJECTIVES

To assess the efficacy of combining daily interruption of sedation with physical and occupational therapy on functional outcomes in patients receiving mechanical ventilation in the ICU.

METHODS

Open label randomized clinical trial on patients receiving sedation and mechanical ventilation at two university hospitals.

Patients

104 mechanically ventilated patients in the ICU received mechanical ventilation for <72 hours, were functionally independent prior to hospitalization, and were expected to continue on the ventilator for at least 24 hours after enrollment.

Interventions

Patients were randomized either to early exercise and mobilization (physical and occupational therapy) during periods of daily interruption of sedation ($n = 49$) or to daily interruption of sedation with therapy as ordered by the primary care team (control, $n = 55$).

Outcomes

The primary outcome was the number of patients returning to independent functional status at hospital discharge. Independent functional status was defined as the ability to perform six activities of daily living and walk independently. The secondary outcomes included duration of delirium and ventilator-free days during the first 28 days of the hospital stay.

KEY RESULTS

- 29 (59%) patients in the intervention group compared to 19 (35%) patients in the control group achieved the primary outcome (return to independent functional status).

- Patients in the intervention group had shorter duration of delirium and more ventilator-free days during the 28-day follow-up period (secondary outcomes).
- There was one serious adverse event in the intervention group (desaturation less than 80%), and discontinuation of therapy as a result of patient instability occurred in 19 (4%) therapy sessions (most commonly for perceived patient–ventilator asynchrony).

STUDY CONCLUSIONS

A program of whole-body rehabilitation including interruption of sedation paired with physical and occupational therapy in the earliest days of critical illness was safe and well tolerated, and resulted in better functional outcomes at hospital discharge, a shorter duration of delirium, and more ventilator-free days compared with standard care.

COMMENTARY

One of the greatest sources of long-term morbidity in the ICU is prolonged immobilization, which often results from sedation-related protocols. In the current study, Schweickert and colleagues hypothesized that early initiation of physical and occupational therapy coupled with daily interruption of sedation would improve functional and neuropsychiatric outcomes. The authors show that early administration of physical therapy (PT) and occupational therapy (OT) in the critical care setting is safe, effective, and improves overall functional independence. This has translated into ICU practice as the push toward earlier physical and occupational therapy protocols. However, patients included in this study were those with independent premorbid functional status and, related to this, were less severely ill (median APACHE II score in the study was 19.5). The generalization of these findings to those with impaired premorbid functioning as well as more critically ill patients remains in question. In addition, although the study claims that there was a reduction in days with delirium in the intervention group, no information is provided regarding assessment of delirium. In summary, this study provides compelling evidence that minimizing sedation and initiating PT and OT as early as possible in the critical care unit improves functional outcomes, but the spectrum of critically ill patients this applies to and the relationship to delirium remain to be answered.

Question

Should minimization of sedation and early PT/OT be pursued in mechanically ventilated patients with critical illness?

Answer

Yes. Minimizing sedation and initiating PT/OT as early as possible improves functional independence.

NEUROINFECTIOUS DISEASES

Jennifer L. Lyons ■ Altaf Saadi

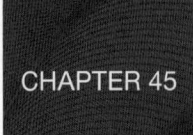

GLUCOCORTICOIDS FOR BACTERIAL MENINGITIS IN ADULTS

CHAPTER 45

Dexamethasone in Adults with Bacterial Meningitis

de Gans J, van de Beek D; European Dexamethasone in Adulthood Bacterial Meningitis Study Investigators. *NEJM*. 2002;347(20):1549–1556

BACKGROUND

Bacterial meningitis is a medical emergency with a high mortality rate if not promptly recognized and treated. Prior to this study, there were sparse and equivocal data on the use of adjuvant corticosteroid therapy in adults with bacterial meningitis.

OBJECTIVES

To determine whether adjunctive dexamethasone treatment improves the outcome of patients with bacterial meningitis.

METHODS

Prospective, randomized, double blind multicenter trial in Amsterdam between June 1993 and December 2001.

Patients

301 patients ages 17 and older were enrolled, with 157 randomized to dexamethasone and 144 to placebo. Patients were included if they had suspected meningitis and a supporting CSF profile. Selected exclusion criteria included those with hypersensitivity to beta-lactam antibiotics or corticosteroids, those treated with antibiotics in the previous 48 hours, and those with history of active tuberculosis or fungal infection.

Interventions

Patients were assigned to receive dexamethasone at a dose of 10 mg every 6 hours intravenously for 4 days, or placebo. The study drug was given before the administration of antibiotics initially, then changed to allow administration of antibiotics concurrently after interim analysis.

Outcomes

Patients were analyzed according to intention to treat. The primary outcome was Glasgow Outcome Scale (GOS) 8 weeks after randomization. Secondary outcome measures were death, focal neurologic abnormalities, hearing loss, gastrointestinal bleeding, fungal infection, herpes zoster, and hyperglycemia.

KEY RESULTS

- Eight weeks after enrollment, an unfavorable outcome defined as moderate or greater disability by the GOS occurred in 15% of the treatment group vs. 25% of the control group (relative risk = 0.59, 95% CI = 0.37–0.94).
- Among the patients with pneumococcal meningitis, 26% in the treatment group had an unfavorable outcome vs. 52% in the placebo group. Among the patients with meningitis because of *Neisseria meningitidis*, there was no significant benefit for adjuvant dexamethasone.
- Seven percent of steroid recipients died vs. 15% of control patients (relative risk = 0.48, 95% CI = 0.24–0.96).
- Focal neurologic deficits and decreased hearing loss showed a trend toward lower frequency in the treatment group than in the control group (13% vs. 20%, p = 0.13 and 9 vs. 12%, p = 0.54, respectively).
- The incidence of adverse effects did not differ between the two groups.

STUDY CONCLUSIONS

Early treatment with dexamethasone reduces the risk of both an unfavorable outcome and death in adults with acute bacterial meningitis. This beneficial effect was not seen on neurologic sequelae, including hearing loss.

COMMENTARY

Following this trial, standard of care now includes prescribing adjunctive cortico-steroids in a suspected bacterial meningitis case. Timing of administration should be before or concurrently with antibiotics. Additionally, most patients in the study received monotherapy with amoxicillin. Currently, there is increased incidence of penicillin-resistant pneumococci, for which combination therapy with vancomycin is recommended. There is theoretical concern that dexamethasone reduces blood–brain permeability and impedes the penetration of vancomycin into the subarach-noid space. Therefore, the findings need to be applied with careful consideration in patients concurrently on vancomycin. Lastly, two points of uncertainty that remain include the duration of dexamethasone and whether corticosteroids are beneficial in significantly immunosuppressed patients with bacterial meningitis. Interestingly, a 2015 Cochrane review of 25 RCT of corticosteroids for acute bacterial meningitis revealed that corticosteroids reduced hearing loss and neurologic sequelae, but overall mortality only in *Streptococcus pneumonia* meningitis.[1] Further, the benefits of cor-ticosteroids were observed in a high-income country setting only, where prevalence of nonpneumococcal meningitis is fewer than in low-income countries.

Question

Should dexamethasone be administered in adults presenting with suspected bacterial meningitis?

Answer

Yes, adults with suspected bacterial meningitis should be started on dexamethasone concurrently with or immediately before the first dose of antibiotics.

Reference

1. Brouwer MC, McIntyer P, Prasad K, et al. Corticosteroids for acute bacterial meningitis. *Cochrane Database Syst Rev.* 2015;(9):CD004405.

CHAPTER 46

ACYCLOVIR FOR HERPES SIMPLEX ENCEPHALITIS

Vidarabine versus Acyclovir Therapy in Herpes Simplex Encephalitis

Whitley RJ, Alford CA, Hirsch MS, et al. *NEJM*. 1986;314(3):144–149

BACKGROUND

Herpes simplex encephalitis (HSE) is recognized worldwide as the most frequent cause of sporadic, often fatal, encephalitis. Before effective antiviral treatment was available, the mortality rate of HSE was about 70%, and most survivors had severe neurologic deficits. This study was the first to report the effectiveness of acyclovir, a selective inhibitor of herpes simplex virus replication, in treating HSE. Before this study, vidarabine was the therapeutic antiviral of choice.

OBJECTIVES

To compare the effectiveness of acyclovir and vidarabine in the treatment of biopsy-proven HSE.

METHODS

A single-blinded randomized controlled multicenter study from 1981 to 1984.

Patients

208 patients, older than 6 months, who underwent brain biopsy for presumptive HSE were randomly assigned to receive either vidarabine or acyclovir. A total of 69 patients had biopsy-proven disease, with 37 randomized to vidarabine and 32 to acyclovir. There were more patients under 30 years of age assigned to the acyclovir group, but in regression analyses, this was not found to influence treatment comparison significantly.

Interventions

Patients received either vidarabine (15 mg/kg of body weight/day) or acyclovir (30 mg/kg/day) for 10 days.

Outcomes

Clinical assessment focused on duration, progression, and severity of disease, particularly the level of consciousness and the GCS score. Mortality at 1 and 6 months and overall (18 months) was assessed for the vidarabine and acyclovir patients. For consistency with the morbidity assessment, 6-month survival was used to determine the factors that influenced outcome. For morbidity, patients were classified at 6 months and beyond as normal; having minor, moderate, or severe impairment; or being dead.

KEY RESULTS

- In biopsy-proven HSE, acyclovir significantly reduced mortality as compared to vidarabine (28% vs. 54%).
- Acyclovir increased the portion of patients with no or mild impairment, as well as those with more severe impairments if they survived.
- Patients under 30 years of age and with a GCS >10 had the best outcome with acyclovir treatment.
- Poor GCS (≤6) at baseline, irrespective of age, was associated with poor outcomes.

STUDY CONCLUSIONS

Acyclovir is the treatment of choice for biopsy-proven HSE, yielding a significant reduction in mortality and morbidity.

COMMENTARY

This trial established the use of acyclovir for the treatment of HSE. The delay in treatment with neurosurgical scheduling, completion of brain biopsy, and resulting pathologic data could have contributed to the deterioration in consciousness of patients and therefore increased mortality or morbidity upon survival in this study. In fact, the disease duration before acyclovir administration was a significant predictor of the mortality in this group (but not in the vidarabine group). Current practice is to initiate therapy as soon as the diagnosis is suspected. Lastly, the duration of the antiviral therapy was ultimately deemed incorrect on follow-up studies. VanLandingham et al.[1] highlighted a case of HSE relapse after a 10-day course of acyclovir therapy, as did several case reports thereafter. Given the low toxic effects of acyclovir and the high morbidity and mortality of HSE, they recommended that all cases be treated with at least 14 to 21 days of acyclovir, which is the treatment duration currently used clinically.

Question

Is acyclovir superior to vidarabine in efficacy as measured by mortality and morbidity?

Answer

Yes, acyclovir reduced mortality and morbidity of patients with HSE and is the recommended therapeutic agent of choice.

Reference

1. VanLandingham KE, Marsteller HB, Ross GW, et al. Relapse of herpes simplex encephalitis after conventional acyclovir therapy. *JAMA*. 1988;259(7):1051–1053.

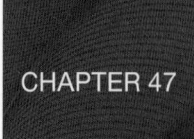

POLYMERASE CHAIN REACTION TESTING FOR HERPES SIMPLEX ENCEPHALITIS

CHAPTER 47

Diagnosis of Herpes Simplex Encephalitis: Application of Polymerase Chain Reaction to Cerebrospinal Fluid from Brain-Biopsied Patients and Correlation with Disease

Lakeman FD, Whitley RJ; National Institute of Allergy and Infectious Diseases Collaborative Antiviral Study Group. *J Infect Dis*. 1995;171(4):857–863

BACKGROUND

At the time of this study, isolation of herpes simplex virus (HSV) from brain tissue after biopsy was the standard for the diagnosis of HSE. At the same time, however, antiviral therapy was known to be most successful if the disease was diagnosed early and treatment initiated early. This study was foundational in establishing polymerase chain reaction (PCR) analyses to detect HSV DNA in CSF specimens.

OBJECTIVES

To develop a sensitive and specific PCR analysis to detect HSV DNA in CSF specimens from patients whose HSE status was based on biopsy.

METHODS

CSF analysis of stored CSF specimens from several studies of biopsy-proven HSE using a novel HSV DNA assay.

Patients

CSF samples from 101 patients were available from prior clinical trials. Of these, 54 patients had biopsy-proven HSE. Patients were classified as biopsy positive or negative on the basis of isolation of HSV from the biopsy specimen in tissue culture.

Interventions

CSF specimens from both biopsy-positive and -negative patients were evaluated with two sets of primers from different regions of the HSV genome. The result from all CSF samples in which HSV DNA was detected using one primer was confirmed using a second set of primers. Inhibition of PCR by a specific CSF sample was also assessed to determine whether negative PCR results indicated a specimen was devoid of HSV DNA or had inhibitory activity.

Outcomes

The sensitivity and specificity of the HSV PCR assay was established among biopsy-proven cases.

KEY RESULTS

- The sensitivity of the PCR assay was 98% and the specificity was 94%.
- The positive and negative predictive values were 95% and 98%, respectively.
- There was no effect of antiviral therapy during the first week of treatment on detection of HSV DNA in the CSF. The effect of antiviral therapy on detection of HSV DNA became evident during the second week of treatment, when only 47% of the specimens remained PCR positive. However, only three of the cases were on acyclovir therapy, with the rest on vidarabine.
- There was no correlation between the persistence of HSV DNA in the CSF with neurologic outcome. Age (older patients) and focal neurologic findings were positively correlated with positive HSV PCR and biopsy-proven disease.

STUDY CONCLUSIONS

The PCR detection of HSV DNA in the CSF is a sensitive and specific method for the diagnosis of HSE.

COMMENTARY

This study established the detection of HSV DNA by CSF PCR as the gold standard for diagnosis, a much more rapid and less invasive HSE detection method than biopsy. In fact, positive PCR results were obtained in three biopsy-negative patients, suggesting that brain biopsy can be fallible, particularly if handled improperly, and PCR may be even superior to biopsy. Other important diagnostic considerations include false-negative results that can occur if CSF samples are obtained early in the course of illness, usually less than 72 hours. Antiviral therapy can decrease the detection of HSV DNA in the CSF of patients, but PCR usually remains positive during the first week of therapy. Further, false-negative results may occur in the setting of a bloody tap or in the presence of xanthochromia. The combination of these findings supports the overall notion that a positive or negative PCR must be interpreted in the context of the clinical presentation, duration of illness, and prior use of antiviral therapy.

Question

Can HSV DNA be detected in the CSF of patients with presumed HSV encephalitis?

Answer

Yes, HSV DNA presence in CSF with PCR method can be detected with high sensitivity and specificity in patients with HSE, making it valid for diagnosis of HSE.

CHAPTER 48

ANTIFUNGAL THERAPY FOR CRYPTOCOCCAL MENINGITIS

Combination Antifungal Therapy for Cryptococcal Meningitis

Day JN, Chau TT, Wobers M, et al. *NEJM*. 2013;368(14):1291–1302

BACKGROUND

The incidence of cryptococcal meningitis (CM) markedly increased as a result of HIV, particularly in developing countries. At the time of this publication, the ideal management of CM remained unclear. Amphotericin B (AmB) and flucytosine had not been shown to reduce mortality as compared to AmB monotherapy, and flucytosine was often not available in areas of the world where disease burden was greatest. Due to greater availability of fluconazole, fluconazole and not flucytosine was part of the treatment regimen for some patients based on their geography.

OBJECTIVES

To determine whether combination induction therapy with either AmB and flucytosine or AmB and fluconazole offered a survival advantage, as compared with AmB alone.

METHODS

Randomized, three-group trial of induction therapy for CM in patients with HIV infection and suspected CM in Ho Chi Minh City, Vietnam, between April 2004 and September 2010.

Patients

299 patients were enrolled and underwent randomization. Inclusion criteria were HIV infection and signs and symptoms of CM (CSF-positive India ink staining, cryptococcal antigen or culture, or blood with positive cryptococcal antigen or culture). Exclusion criteria included having received antifungal therapy for more than 3 days, pregnancy, renal or liver failure, or concurrent rifampin use.

Interventions

100 patients were assigned to receive AmB (1 mg/kg/day) for 4 weeks; 100 patients were assigned to receive AmB and flucytosine (100 mg/kg/day) for 2 weeks; 99 were assigned to receive AmB and fluconazole (400 mg twice daily) for 2 weeks. After induction therapy, patients received oral fluconazole for a total of a 10-week treatment course. lumbar punctures (LPs) were performed weekly for the first month of treatment and then as clinically indicated. Patients were assessed monthly for 6 months.

Outcomes

Coprimary outcomes were all-cause mortality in the first 14 and 70 days after randomization. Secondary outcomes were mortality at 6 months, disability status at 70 days and

6 months, changes in CSF fungal counts in first 2 weeks, time to CSF sterilization, and adverse events during the first 10 weeks of the study.

KEY RESULTS
- Combination therapy with AmB and flucytosine was associated with improved survival both at 10 weeks (HR = 0.61, 95% CI = 0.39–0.97, p = 0.04) and at 6 months (HR = 0.56, 95% CI = 0.36–0.86), as compared with AmB monotherapy.
- Combination therapy with AmB and flucytosine was also associated with a significantly higher chance of being free of disability at 6 months than those receiving monotherapy.
- The time to fungal clearance was significantly shorter in patients receiving AmB plus flucytosine than in the other groups.
- Adverse events were similar in all treatment groups.

STUDY CONCLUSIONS
AmB plus flucytosine is associated with improved survival and disability status among patients with CM, as compared with AmB monotherapy. No survival benefit for AmB plus fluconazole was found.

COMMENTARY

This study established the recommended induction treatment for CM as a combination of AmB and flucytosine, which confers both a mortality and morbidity benefit compared to both AmB and fluconazole and AmB monotherapy. Importantly, not all patients in this study were on antiretroviral therapy (ART). The study therefore could not determine whether ART improved survival, or if manifestation of immune reconstitution inflammatory syndrome (IRIS) could have worsened it. Regardless, given the survival benefit of adding flucytosine to AmB for treating CM, this study led support to efforts in improving access to flucytosine in resource-limited settings.

Question

Is there a survival benefit to AmB and flucytosine combination induction therapy among patients with HIV-associated CM?

Answer

Yes, AmB and flucytosine combination therapy improves survival and disability status as compared to AmB monotherapy or AmB and fluconazole combination therapy.

CHAPTER 49

GUIDELINES FOR TREATMENT OF LYME DISEASE IN THE NERVOUS SYSTEM

Practice Parameter: Treatment of Nervous System Lyme Disease (An Evidence-Based Review): Report of the Quality Standards Subcommittee of the American Academy of Neurology

Halperin JJ, Shapiro ED, Logigian E, et al. *Neurology.* 2007;69(1):91–102

BACKGROUND

Lyme neuroborreliosis (LNB) is neurologic involvement secondary to Lyme disease. This report by the Quality Standards Subcommittee of the American Academy of Neurology attempted to address controversy that existed in the diagnosis and treatment of LNB, because of the wide spectrum of clinical signs and symptoms and competing evidence about use and duration of parenteral vs. oral antibiotics.

OBJECTIVES

To provide evidence-based recommendations on the treatment of CNS Lyme, with regard to (1) which antimicrobial agents are effective; (2) the different regiments preferred for different manifestations of nervous system Lyme disease; and (3) optimal duration of therapy needed.

METHODS

An expert panel of investigators from the United States and Europe was convened. In May 2004, an Ovid MEDLINE, PubMed, and EMBASE literature search (all languages) was performed. Articles were excluded if they did not address treatment of LNB, were not peer reviewed, or were solely review articles. Studies were graded as Class I through IV using standard criteria, and recommendations were made according to review of this data.

Patients
NA

Interventions
NA

Outcomes
An initial 353 citations was reduced to 112 articles after removing duplications. The panel added 10 additional articles. After detailed review of the 122 articles, the panel decided 37 articles contributed relevant data. Four studies were Class I. Four studies were Class II. The remainder of studies were Class III or IV.

KEY RESULTS
- Lyme disease involving the nervous system responds well to penicillin, ceftriaxone, cefotaxime, and doxycycline based on four Class II studies.

- The use of oral doxycycline for central nervous system (CNS) Lyme disease is comparable to IV antibiotic regimens because of excellent CSF penetration achieved by doxycycline. This is supported by two Class II studies and numerous Class III and IV studies. There is a low probability of neurologic sequelae after doxycycline treatment.
- For parenchymal involvement or severe neurologic symptoms, parenteral antibiotic regimens may be associated with better outcomes than oral regimens based on one Class I and one Class II study.
- For both oral and parenteral regimens, the recommended duration is 14 days. Some studies using courses from 10 to 28 days did not reveal significantly different outcomes.
- Post-Lyme syndrome does not respond to prolonged courses of antibiotics (of up to 12 weeks) based on three randomized, double-blind, placebo-controlled trials.

STUDY CONCLUSIONS

(1) Parenteral penicillin, ceftriaxone, and cefotaxime are safe and effective treatment for peripheral and CNS Lyme disease (Level B); (2) oral doxycycline is safe and effective for peripheral and CNS Lyme disease (Level B); and (3) prolonged courses of antibiotics do not improve outcome of post-Lyme syndrome and are not recommended (Level A).

COMMENTARY

By reviewing and classifying available data based on the rigor of research (Class I to Class IV), these guidelines help practitioners make evidence-based clinical decisions. Namely, LNB can respond well to multiple antibiotics, and outcomes may be comparable between oral and parenteral regimens in the absence of brain or spinal cord involvement or severe neurologic symptoms. The duration of treatment is recommended to be 14 days, with no benefit for prolonged antibiotics including for post-Lyme syndrome. It is important to note that the oral antibiotic data are entirely from Europe. Although European Lyme strains are similar to North American strains, they are not identical. Subsequently, findings are sometimes applied with caution when applied to North American context.

Question

Is there data to support the use of oral vs. parenteral antibiotics for CNS Lyme?

Answer

Yes, there is evidence to support the use of both oral and parenteral antibiotics for CNS Lyme, although in the United States, CNS Lyme is preferentially treated with ceftriaxone.

SECTION 6

NEURO-ONCOLOGY

Mikael L. Rinne ■ Maya Srikanth Graham

CHAPTER 50

TEMOZOLOMIDE FOR GLIOBLASTOMA

Radiotherapy Plus Concomitant and Adjuvant Temozolomide for Glioblastoma

Stupp R, Mason WP, van den Bent MJ, et al. *NEJM*. 2005;352:987–996

BACKGROUND
Glioblastoma (GBM) is a primary malignant brain tumor with a dismal prognosis. Median survival in 2005 was less than 1 year, with standard treatment consisting of maximal safe surgical resection followed by radiation. At that time, no phase III trials had demonstrated a survival benefit from chemotherapy. This study was the first in GBM to demonstrate a clear survival benefit from temozolomide.

OBJECTIVES
To evaluate the efficacy of combination radiation therapy and temozolomide in the treatment of GBM.

METHODS
International randomized controlled trial across 85 centers from 2000 to 2002.

Patients
573 patients with newly diagnosed GBM between ages 18 and 70, with adequate performance status as well as hematologic, renal, and hepatic function. Patients were centrally randomized within 6 weeks of diagnosis and must have been on stable or decreasing doses of corticosteroids for the preceding 2 weeks.

Interventions
Standard focal radiation therapy (RT; 60 Gy fractionated over 30 sessions; control group) vs. radiation with concomitant daily temozolomide (75 mg/m^2) followed by 6 monthly cycles of adjuvant temozolomide (starting at 150 mg/m^2 and increasing to 200 mg/m^2 as tolerated).

Outcomes
The primary end point was overall survival (OS). Secondary end points were progression-free survival (PFS), safety, and quality of life (reported separately).

KEY RESULTS

- Addition of temozolomide to radiation increased median OS (14.6 months, 95% CI = 13.2–16.8) compared with radiation alone (12.1 months, 95% CI = 11.2–13.0).
- Median PFS with radiation plus temozolomide was 6.9 months (95% CI = 5.8–8.2) compared with 5.0 months with radiation alone (95% CI = 4.2–5.5).
- Temozolomide was associated with an increase in grade 3 and 4 hematologic toxicities (21%) compared to none in the radiation alone arm.

STUDY CONCLUSIONS

Addition of concomitant and adjuvant temozolomide to RT provides a clinically meaningful increase in survival for GBM patients.

COMMENTARY

This was the first phase III study in GBMs to evaluate combination therapy and showed a clinically significant improvement in survival with the addition of temozolomide. This led to a new standard of care for treating GBMs. Subsequent analyses showed that patients with GBM containing a methylated O^6-methylguanine-DNA methyltransferase (MGMT) promoter were more likely to benefit from temozolomide.[1] It should be noted that patients in the control arm of the study had prolonged survival as compared with historical controls, perhaps due to the inclusion criteria regarding age and performance status, which may limit its applicability to patients who are older or more ill at the time of diagnosis.

Question

Does addition of temozolomide to radiotherapy improve survival in GBM?

Answer

Yes, temozolomide when combined with radiation improves OS by 2.5 months.

Reference

1. Hegi ME, Diserens AC, Gorlia T, et al. MGMT gene silencing and benefit from temozolomide in glioblastoma. *NEJM*. 2005;352(10):997–1003.

CHAPTER 51

SURGERY FOR BRAIN METASTASES

A Randomized Trial of Surgery in the Treatment of Single Metastases to the Brain
Patchell RA, Tibbs PA, Walsh JW, et al. *NEJM*. 1990;322:494–500

BACKGROUND

Brain metastases are the most common intracranial tumor, and, at the time of this 1990 study, were associated with a median survival of less than 6 months. Standard of care at the time was whole brain RT alone, even though approximately 50% of brain metastases are single masses that may be amenable to surgical resection. No controlled clinical trials had been performed to assess the potential benefit of surgical resection in patients with single brain metastases.

OBJECTIVES

To assess the potential benefit of surgical resection in the management of single brain metastases.

METHODS

Randomized single-center controlled trial from October 1985 to December 1988.

Patients

48 patients with radiographic evidence of single brain metastasis with histologic confirmation of a systemic cancer within 5 years. Patients were excluded if their lesions were not surgically resectable or if they were known to have a particularly radiosensitive primary cancer (i.e., small cell lung cancer, germ-cell tumors, lymphoma, leukemia, and multiple myeloma).

Interventions

Whole brain RT (36 Gy in 3 Gy fractions) after either supratentorial stereotactic biopsy (radiation group) or gross total resection (surgery group). Biopsy or resection was performed within 72 hours of diagnosis, followed by radiation within 48 hours of biopsy or 14 days of resection.

Outcomes

Time to recurrence of brain metastasis, OS, functional independence (indicated by Karnofsky Performance Score $\geq$70), and mortality because of neurologic complications (neurologic survival).

KEY RESULTS

- Surgical resection followed by radiation improves median survival (40 weeks) as compared to radiation alone (15 weeks, $p < 0.01$); relative risk of death 2.2 (95% CI = 1.2–4.1).

- Surgical resection reduces the incidence of local recurrence (20% vs. 52%, $p < 0.02$) and increases the time to local recurrence (>59 weeks vs. 21 weeks, $p < 0.001$) as compared with radiation alone.
- Neurologic survival was also improved with surgical resection (62 weeks) compared with radiation alone (26 weeks, $p < 0.0009$), relative risk of neurologic death 5.2 (95% CI = 1.8–15.2).
- Duration of functional independence was increased with surgical resection (38 weeks) compared with radiation alone (8 weeks, $p < 0.005$), relative risk 2.4 (95% CI = 1.3–4.6).
- 30-Day mortality was identical between the two groups (4%).

STUDY CONCLUSIONS

Surgical resection prior to whole brain RT improves the survival and quality of life of patients with single brain metastases.

COMMENTARY

Surgery in these patients was not routinely considered prior to this study, but as a result of these findings became standard of care. Interestingly, this study also demonstrated the importance of a tissue diagnosis in patients with single brain lesions in the setting of systemic cancer, as an additional 11% of patients initially suspected of having brain metastasis were found not to have intracranial metastases upon biopsy. Patchell and colleagues subsequently studied the efficacy of postoperative radiotherapy after complete surgical resection and found that patients who received whole brain radiotherapy following complete resection had significantly lower recurrence rates than those treated with surgery alone, although OS was unchanged.[1] Patchell and colleagues also subsequently demonstrated that decompressive surgery plus postoperative radiotherapy was superior to radiotherapy alone for treatment of spinal cord compression caused by metastatic cancer.[2]

Question

Is there a role for surgery in the management of brain metastases?

Answer

Yes, surgical resection of single brain metastases followed by whole brain RT improves OS and functional independence compared with radiation alone.

References

1. Patchell RA, Tibbs PA, Regine WF, et al. Postoperative radiotherapy in the treatment of single metastases to the brain: a randomized trial. *JAMA.* 1998;280(17):1485–1489.
2. Patchell RA, Tibbs PA, Regine WF, et al. Direct decompressive surgical resection in the treatment of spinal cord compression caused by metastatic cancer: a randomised trial. *Lancet.* 2005;366(9486):643–648.

CHAPTER 52

CHEMOTHERAPY FOR LOW-GRADE GLIOMA

Radiation Plus Procarbazine, CCNU and Vincristine in Low-Grade Glioma

Buckner JC, Shaw EG, Pugh SL, et al. *NEJM*. 2016;374(14):1344–1355

BACKGROUND

Low-grade gliomas (LGGs) are infiltrative tumors that most often afflict young adults and lead to neurologic decline and premature death. Prior studies had established standard of care as maximal safe surgical resection followed by radiotherapy, but the benefit of chemotherapy remained unclear.

OBJECTIVES

To assess the potential benefit of adjuvant chemotherapy following surgery and radiation in LGGs.

METHODS

Randomized multicenter controlled trial from 1998 to 2002.

Patients

251 patients with supratentorial histologically proven WHO Grade II astrocytomas, oligodendrogliomas, or mixed oligoastrocytomas. Only high-risk patients were included, defined as ages 18 to 39 years with subtotal resection or age greater than 40 years with gross total resection. Exclusion criteria included alternate pathologies on central histology review, noncontiguous leptomeningeal spread of disease, gliomatosis cerebri, synchronous or prior systemic malignancy (unless disease-free for 5 years), and prior radiation/chemotherapy.

Interventions

Tumor-focused fractionated RT (54 Gy over 30 fractions in 6 weeks) with or without 6 cycles of postradiation procarbazine, lomustine, and vincristine (RT+PCV, 8 weeks/cycle).

Outcomes

The primary endpoint was OS. PFS was the secondary endpoint.

KEY RESULTS

- There was an improvement in median OS with RT+PCV (13.3 years, 95% CI = 10.6–not reached) as compared with RT alone (7.8 years, 95% CI = 6.1–9.8), HR = 0.59, p = 0.003.

- There was an increase in PFS with RT+PCV (10.4 years, 95% CI = 6.1–not reached) compared to RT alone (4.0 years, 95% CI = 3.1–5.5), HR = 0.50, $p < 0.001$.
- The rate of PFS at 10 years was 51% in the RT+PCV group (95% CI = 42%–59%) vs. 21% in the RT alone group (95% CI = 14%–28%).

STUDY CONCLUSIONS

Adjuvant RT+PCV chemotherapy increases both OS and PFS in patients with high-risk LGGs (patients older than 40 years or those with incompletely resected tumors).

COMMENTARY

Standard of care for LGGs prior to this study was maximal safe resection followed by RT, though timing of radiation (early vs. delayed) was unclear.[1] Preliminary data from this study published in 2012 provided the first randomized controlled evidence of an improvement in PFS, although there was no difference in OS at that time. The current study includes long-term follow-up demonstrating a near doubling of OS. Importantly, *IDH1* mutation status could only be evaluated in approximately 45% of patients, and 1p19q codeletion was not assessed. Although not sufficiently powered for subgroup analyses, the magnitude of benefit was greatest for oligodendrogliomas and IDH1 mutant tumors. After this study completed enrollment, temozolomide was demonstrated to prolong OS in patients with GBM. This study does not address the efficacy of temozolomide for LGGs.

Question

Is there a role for chemotherapy in the treatment of LGGs?

Answer

Yes, PCV-based chemotherapy improves both overall and PFS following surgery and RT in the treatment of LGGs.

Reference

1. van den Bent MJ, Afra D, de Witte O, et al. Long-term efficacy of early versus delayed radiotherapy for low-grade astrocytoma and oligodendroglioma in adults: the EORTC 22845 randomised trial. *Lancet.* 2005;366(9490):985–990.

CHAPTER 53

NovoTTF FOR NEWLY DIAGNOSED GLIOBLASTOMA

Maintenance Therapy with Tumor-Treating Fields Plus Temozolomide vs Temozolomide Alone for Glioblastoma: A Randomized Clinical Trial

Stupp R, Taillibert S, Kanner AA, et al. *JAMA*. 2015;314(23):2535–2543

BACKGROUND

Despite the improvement in OS with the addition of temozolomide, median survival for GBM has remained less than 2 years for more than a decade. Tumor-treating fields (TTFields) are a novel therapeutic strategy that utilizes alternating electric fields to inhibit tumor proliferation. Preclinical studies have shown that TTFields disrupt mitotic spindle formation, causing mitotic arrest and apoptosis. A previous randomized phase III trial showed quality of life benefits in recurrent GBM; however, PFS and OS were not improved.[1]

OBJECTIVES

To evaluate the efficacy and safety of TTFields in combination with temozolomide in newly diagnosed GBM patients after standard initial chemoradiation therapy.

METHODS

Open-label, randomized multicenter international controlled trial between 2009 and 2014.

Patients

695 patients (315 included in primary interim analysis) with newly diagnosed supratentorial GBM and adequate performance status who completed initial temozolomide/RT. Exclusion criteria included progression of disease prior to randomization and severe comorbidities.

Interventions

Patients were randomized 2:1 to standard adjuvant temozolomide for 6 to 12 cycles with or without continuous TTFields treatment (worn for at least 18 hours/day). TTFields could be continued until second progression or clinical decline for a maximum of 24 months.

Outcomes

The primary outcome was PFS in the intent-to-treat population. The secondary endpoint was OS in the per-protocol population.

KEY RESULTS

- Median PFS was improved in the TTFields group (7.1 months, 95% CI = 5.9–8.2) compared with the temozolomide alone group (4.0 months, 95% CI = 3.3–5.2), HR = 0.62, 95% CI = 0.43–0.89, $p = 0.001$.

- OS in the per-protocol population was improved in the TTFields group (20.5 months, 95% CI = 16.7–25.0) compared with the temozolomide alone group (15.6 months, 95% CI = 13.3–19.1), HR = 0.64, 95% CI = 0.42–0.98, p = 0.004.
- OS and 2-year survival in the intent-to-treat population were also significantly increased.
- There was no significant increase in systemic toxic effects with TTFields (mild skin reactions, confusion, headaches were more common in the TTFields group).

STUDY CONCLUSIONS

The addition of TTFields to adjuvant temozolomide improves both OS and PFS in GBM patients without significant adverse effects.

COMMENTARY

This study validated TTFields as a viable and well-tolerated treatment modality that significantly improves survival in GBM patients. Of note, patients with progression of disease after diagnosis but before randomization (an average period of 3.8 months) were excluded from this study. As such, the study results may not be applicable to patients with more aggressive clinical courses. Efficacy is also dependent on compliance with treatment protocol (must shave head and wear device, attached to a battery pack, for ≥18 hours/day).

Question

Are there any treatments that improve survival in GBM beyond standard chemoradiation?

Answer

Yes, treatment with TTFields in combination with standard chemoradiation therapy yields a significant improvement in survival in patients with GBM.

Reference

1. Stupp R, Wong ET, Kanner AA, et al. NovoTTF-100A versus physician's choice chemotherapy in recurrent glioblastoma: a randomised phase III trial of a novel treatment modality. *Eur J Cancer.* 2012;48(14):2192–2202.

CHAPTER 54

BEVACIZUMAB FOR RECURRENT GLIOBLASTOMA

Bevacizumab Alone and in Combination with Irinotecan in Recurrent Glioblastoma
Friedman HS, Prados MD, Wen PY, et al. *J Clin Oncol*. 2009;27(28):4733

BACKGROUND
Although the introduction of temozolomide significantly impacted the treatment of newly diagnosed GBM, tumor relapse is inevitable. Therapeutic strategies for recurrent GBM have not been standardized, and at the time of this study, most providers turned to cytotoxic agents such as irinotecan with limited success (6 months PFS 9% to 21%).

OBJECTIVES
To evaluate the efficacy of the anti–vascular endothelial growth factor (VEGF) antibody bevacizumab alone or in addition to irinotecan in the treatment of recurrent GBM.

METHODS
Multicenter, open-label, noncomparative phase II trial from 2006 to 2007.

Patients
167 patients with histologically confirmed recurrent GBM (first or second recurrence) with evidence of disease progression on MRI within 2 weeks of study drug initiation. Notable exclusion criteria included prior treatment with similar agents, recent intracranial hemorrhage, prior coagulopathy or bleeding diathesis, arterial thromboembolism within the prior 6 months, or significant cardiovascular disease (including uncontrolled hypertension).

Interventions
Patients were randomized to bevacizumab or bevacizumab plus irinotecan. Bevacizumab was given every other week for a total of 104 weeks or until evidence of disease progression. Radiographic evaluation was blinded.

Outcomes
The primary outcomes were 6 months PFS (PFS6) and objective response rates (OR, defined as stable to improved consecutive MRIs ≥4 weeks apart). Secondary outcomes were OS, PFS, and response duration.

KEY RESULTS
- PFS6 rates were 42.6% (97.5% CI = 29.6%–55.5%) with bevacizumab and 50.3% (97.5% CI = 36.8%–63.9%) with bevacizumab + irinotecan; $p < 0.0001$ compared to assumed 6-month PFS of 15% for salvage chemotherapy or irinotecan alone.

- OR rate 28.2% (97.5% CI = 18.5%–40.3%) with bevacizumab and 37.8% (97.5% CI = 26.5%–50.8%) with bevacizumab + irinotecan; $p < 0.0001$ compared to assumed OR rate of 5% for salvage chemotherapy and 10% for irinotecan alone.
- The most common significant adverse events were hypertension and convulsion in the bevacizumab group compared to convulsion, neutropenia, and fatigue in the bevacizumab + irinotecan group. Notable additional adverse events in the bevacizumab group included both arterial and venous thromboembolism.

STUDY CONCLUSIONS

Bevacizumab demonstrates substantial antitumor activity in recurrent GBM patients, both alone and in combination with irinotecan, far exceeding historical controls for salvage chemotherapy in terms of progression free survival. Though there were significant adverse events, they were in keeping with prior studies of these agents in other patient populations.

COMMENTARY

This study was the first large trial to explore the potential utility of antiangiogenic therapy with the VEGF inhibitor bevacizumab in patients with recurrent GBM. A single-arm study published in the same year showed similar response rates and improvement in PFS.[1] Bevacizumab was subsequently approved by the Food and Drug Administration (FDA) for treatment of recurrent GBM in 2009 and has been widely adopted for the treatment of recurrent GBM in the United States. However, it should be noted that as bevacizumab targets neoangiogenesis, its effect as measured by contrast extravasation on MRI may be out of proportion to its actual antitumor activity; some studies have shown that bevacizumab may be associated with more nonenhancing progression. Multiple phase III studies have since failed to demonstrate an OS advantage of bevacizumab in patients with newly diagnosed[2,3] and recurrent GBM.[4]

Question

Is there a role for targeted antiangiogenic therapies such as bevacizumab in the treatment of recurrent GBM?

Answer

Probably. Bevacizumab provides a notable improvement in PFS in patients with recurrent GBM with tolerable adverse events, although emerging evidence appears to indicate no effect on OS.

References

1. Kreisl TN, Kim L, Moore K, et al. Phase II trial of single-agent bevacizumab followed by bevacizumab plus irinotecan at tumor progression in recurrent glioblastoma. *J Clin Oncol.* 2009;27(5):740–745.
2. Chinot OL, Wick W, Mason W, et al. Bevacizumab plus radiotherapy-temozolomide for newly diagnosed glioblastoma. *NEJM.* 2014;370(8):709–722.
3. Gilbert MR, Dignam JJ, Armstrong TS, et al. A randomized trial of bevacizumab for newly diagnosed glioblastoma. *NEJM.* 2014;370(8):699–708.
4. Wick W, Brandes A, Gorlia T, et al. Phase III trial exploring the combination of bevacizumab and lomustine in patients with first recurrence of a glioblastoma: the EORTC 26101 trial. *Neuro-Oncol.* 2015;17(suppl 5):v1.5–v1.

CHAPTER 55

METHOTREXATE FOR PRIMARY CNS LYMPHOMA

Treatment of Primary CNS Lymphoma with Methotrexate and Deferred Radiotherapy: A Report of NABTT 96-07

Batchelor T, Carson K, O'Neill A, et al. *J Clin Oncol*. 2003;21(6):1044

BACKGROUND

Primary CNS lymphoma (PCNSL) is an uncommon non-Hodgkin lymphoma, typically of the diffuse large B-cell subtype, that is restricted to the CNS. Attempts to extrapolate treatment strategies used in systemic lymphomas (such as R-CHOP) have been limited in part by the blood–brain barrier, and whole-brain radiation therapy (WBRT) is both unable to establish a durable response and is also fraught with neurocognitive side effects, particularly in the elderly. A contemporary retrospective study published in 2002 showed that treatment with chemoradiation was superior to radiation alone, and patients who received high-dose methotrexate had improved survival compared to other drugs.[1]

OBJECTIVES

To determine if high-dose methotrexate monotherapy of PCNSL is of comparable efficacy to historical results of more toxic chemotherapeutic regimens.

METHODS

Phase II multicenter open-label noncomparative trial from 1998 to 1999.

Patients

25 patients with newly diagnosed, pathologically confirmed PCNSL with sufficient performance status and renal function. Notable exclusion criteria included HIV seropositivity and evidence of systemic lymphoma.

Interventions

Induction (every 2 weeks until complete response [CR] or 8 cycles total), consolidation (2 additional 2 week cycles) and maintenance (11 cycles every 4 weeks) methotrexate treatment. Each treatment cycle required hospital admission for IV hydration and urine alkalinization with sodium bicarbonate, as well as leucovorin rescue monitored by methotrexate level.

Outcomes

The primary outcomes were radiographic CR or partial response (PR). Secondary outcomes included OS and PFS, and patients were additionally monitored for drug-related toxicity.

KEY RESULTS

- 52% of patients demonstrated a CR and 22% demonstrated a PR (total response rate 74%), whereas 22% demonstrated progression during treatment. 22% of patients exhibited a durable remission of >2 years.
- Median PFS was 12.8 months; median OS had not yet been reached in the nearly 2 years of follow-up.
- 52% of patients experienced grade 3 or 4 toxicities, although not all of these were thought to be related to methotrexate treatment.
- There was minimal decline in cognitive status with methotrexate treatment, as measured by longitudinal Mini-Mental State Examination (MMSE).

STUDY CONCLUSIONS

High-dose methotrexate monotherapy is a feasible approach to PCNSL treatment with meaningful response rates and modest toxicities.

COMMENTARY

Standard of care for PCNSL patients at the time of this trial consisted of multi-drug regimens combined with whole-brain radiotherapy, which often resulted in significant delayed neurotoxicity. This study laid the groundwork for establishing high-dose methotrexate as an efficacious treatment that allowed for the deferral of RT, vastly improving the toxicity profile of treatment. It is important to note that this was not an RCT, so historical controls were used for comparison. In addition, the median follow-up time was about 2 years, which may not be sufficient to reveal potential delayed neurotoxicity from treatment or late relapses. Finally, this was a small study of only 25 patients. Subsequently published final results from a phase II trial in newly diagnosed PCNSL patients of high-dose methotrexate with or without whole-brain radiotherapy at relapse showed only modest efficacy of combined therapy, but confirmed a significantly higher incidence of leukoencephalopathy in patients who underwent WBRT.[2]

Question

Does high-dose methotrexate yield meaningful responses in the treatment of PCNSL?

Answer

Yes, methotrexate monotherapy results in substantial clinical response with a reduced toxicity profile compared to contemporary regimens including whole-brain radiotherapy.

References

1. Ferreri AJ, Reni M, Pasini F, et al. A multicenter study of treatment of primary CNS lymphoma. *Neurology.* 2002;58(10):1513–1520.
2. Herrlinger U, Kuker W, Uhl M, et al. NOA-03 trial of high-dose methotrexate in primary central nervous system lymphoma: final report. *Ann Neurol.* 2005;57(6):843–847.

NEUROMUSCULAR

Michael P. Bowley ■ Kathleen E. McKee

CHAPTER 56

ACUTE TREATMENT FOR GUILLAIN–BARRE SYNDROME

Randomised Trial of Plasma Exchange, Intravenous Immunoglobulin, and Combined Treatments in Guillain-Barre Syndrome

Plasma Exchange/Sandoglobulin Guillain-Barre Syndrome Trial Group. *Lancet.* 1997;349(9047):225–230

BACKGROUND

Guillain–Barre syndrome (GBS) most commonly manifests as an acute monophasic paralyzing illness. Pathogenesis is thought to be an autoimmune response usually provoked by a preceding infection. Despite its autoimmune etiology and similarity to chronic inflammatory demyelinating polyneuropathy (which does respond to steroids) prior studies have demonstrated steroids are ineffective in treating acute GBS.[1] Both plasma exchange (PE) and IVIg are known to accelerate recovery, but their relative efficacy was unknown.

OBJECTIVES

To determine whether IVIg is equivalent to or superior to PE in the treatment of GBS, and whether PE followed by IVIg is superior to single treatment.

METHODS

RCT at 38 centers in 11 countries between January 1993 and April 1995.

Patients

383 patients with severe GBS (requiring aid to walk or worse) with onset of symptoms within the previous 14 days were randomized. Patients with atypical forms of GBS, serious preexisting other disease, or contraindications to PE or IVIg were excluded.

Interventions

Patients were randomized to receive one of three treatment courses: (1) five 50 mL/kg PEs during the 8 to 13 days after randomization; (2) 0.4 g/kg of human immunoglobulin (Sandoglobulin, Sandoz, Basel, Switzerland) daily for 5 days; (3) five 50 mL/kg PEs followed by Sandoglobulin 0.4 g/kg daily for 5 days starting on the day after the last PE.

Outcomes

Primary outcome was difference in the mean improvement in disability grade after 4 weeks between the two groups (IVIg vs. PE; PE followed by IVIg vs. the better single treatment). Secondary outcome measures were time from randomization to unaided walking, time to permanent discontinuation of artificial ventilation, and average rate of recovery derived from the changes in disability grade over the 48-week follow-up period.

KEY RESULTS

- There were no significant differences between the groups in the major outcome criterion, the mean disability grade improvement after 4 weeks.
- There were no significant differences between groups in any of the secondary outcome criteria.
- There were no significant differences in the numbers of side effects attributed to the treatments.
- 2.3% of patients received less than the planned 75% of the IVIg treatment. 13.8% of patients received less than the 75% of planned PE treatment.

STUDY CONCLUSIONS

IVIg is equivalent to PE in reducing the amount of disability at 4 weeks in GBS. The combined regimen of PE followed by IVIg is not significantly superior to either single treatment modality.

COMMENTARY

This study compared IVIg vs. PE vs. a combined regimen of PE followed immediately by IVIg and found no significant difference between any of these three treatment modalities with respect to disability at 4 weeks or any of the secondary outcome measures. Although there were no significant differences in the numbers of side effects attributed to the treatments, there was one patient death attributed to PE. Additionally, a higher percentage of patients (in this and prior trials) did not complete the entire planned PE course due to complications with the therapy. Because IVIg has now been shown to be of equal therapeutic benefit to PE and is a simpler, more comfortable, and a possibly safer treatment that is more likely to be administered in its entirety, it may be the preferred initial treatment modality in acute GBS.

Question

Is IVIg equivalent to PE in reducing disability at 4 weeks in GBS?

Answer

Yes, this trial demonstrates IVIg is noninferior to PE. Additionally, the combined regimen of PE followed by IVIg is not superior to either agent administered as monotherapy.

Reference

1. Guillain-Barre Syndrome Steroid Trial Group. Double-blind trial of intravenous methylprednisolone in Guillan-Barre syndrome. *Lancet.* 1993;341(8845):586–590.

ALTERNATE DAY PREDNISONE IN MYASTHENIA GRAVIS

Benefit from Alternate-Day Prednisone in Myasthenia Gravis

Warmolts JR, Engel WK. *NEJM*. 1972;286:17–20

BACKGROUND

Myasthenia gravis (MG) is an autoimmune disorder affecting the neuromuscular junction. Acetylcholinesterase inhibitors were serendipitously discovered in the 1930s to provide symptomatic benefit, but prior to the 1970s no disease-modifying treatments had been clearly identified. At the time of this study, it was not known if oral corticosteroids provided benefit to adult patients with MG.

OBJECTIVES

To trial alternate-day prednisone therapy in adult patients with MG with the aim of suppressing a "theoretical immunologic or chemical insult" against the lower motor neuron or inducing a direct or indirect improvement on lower motor neuron function (of note, this study preceded the discovery of the role of postsynaptic acetylcholine receptors in MG).

METHODS

Case series of five adults with MG treated with long-term prednisone and followed for 6 to 17 months at the National Institutes of Health in 1970 to 1971.

Patients

5 adults with MG of varying severity and duration. Electromyography, muscle biopsy, serum enzymes, and other studies were utilized to exclude diseases known to present with myasthenic features.

Interventions

Patients were hospitalized and all anticholinesterase medication was stopped. Prednisone was initiated as an 8 a.m. single 100 mg dose every other day in conjunction with daily potassium supplements and antacids. After improvement and stabilization, patients were discharged and prednisone was continued for greater than 6 months with dose adjustments for some patients.

Outcomes

All patients were monitored for acute and long-term clinical improvement in strength. Some patients were monitored with serial nerve conduction studies acutely.

KEY RESULTS

- Clinical improvement in muscle function appeared 24 to 72 hours after initiation of prednisone therapy.

- Acutely, a 48-hour cyclic improvement of muscle strength and endurance was demonstrated with nerve conduction studies on some patients, and noted to correlate with prednisone administration.
- Improvement was maintained from 6 to 17 months.
- Complete remission of symptoms was obtained in one patient in 4 months and maintained for 13 months.

STUDY CONCLUSIONS

Benefit observed in these five patients was attributed to prednisone. The 48-hour cyclic improvement was in phase with prednisone administration alone and thus not attributed to potassium administration, anticholinesterase withdrawal, or bed rest. Each patient made steady improvement and ultimately achieved a functional level surpassing that previously achieved with cholinesterase inhibitors.

COMMENTARY

In the 1970s MG was still a severely debilitating and sometimes fatal disease. The prior use of oral corticosteroids in MG had received sparse and unfavorable attention aside from a 1971 case series from Denmark reporting almost complete remission in six of seven patients.[1] This 1972 case series by Warmolts and Engel, although small, was a landmark study because of its design. It eliminated the variable of anticholinesterase inhibitors during prednisone initiation—a variable that may have confounded prior studies. Additionally, through correlating spaced administration of prednisone with improvement on serial nerve conduction studies, it provided a convincing link between prednisone and clinical improvement. This study ushered in an era of disease-modifying treatment for MG. Steroids were followed by the discovery of other immunosuppressive drugs for chronic treatment and utilization of plasmapheresis and IV immune globulin for acute exacerbations.

Question

Does oral prednisone for patients with MG provide acute and sustained clinical benefit?

Answer

Yes, oral prednisone correlated with marked improvement in weakness, resulting in a return to functional living for previous severely debilitated patients.

Reference

1. Kjaer M. Myasthenia gravis and myasthenic syndromes treated with prednisone. *Acta Neurol Scand.* 1971;47:464–474.

CHAPTER 58

IVIg VS. PREDNISONE FOR CHRONIC INFLAMMATORY DEMYELINATING POLYNEUROPATHY

Randomized Controlled Trial of Intravenous Immunoglobulin versus Oral Prednisolone in Chronic Inflammatory Demyelinating Polyradiculoneuropathy

Hughes R, Bensa S, Willison H, et al. *Ann Neurol.* 2001;50(2):195–201

BACKGROUND

Chronic inflammatory demyelinating polyradiculoneuropathy (CIDP) is characterized by progressive or relapsing weakness attributed to a demyelinating polyradiculoneuropathy with evidence of slowing or conduction block on nerve conduction studies. An immunologic cause is strongly suspected, and randomized trials have established short-term response to immunomodulatory therapy with glucocorticoids, IV immune globulin (IVIg), or PE.

OBJECTIVES

To determine whether a standard IVIg regimen is more efficacious than a standard oral steroid regimen in CIDP.

METHODS

Randomized, double-blind, crossover trial conducted at nine European centers between July 1998 and November 1999.

Patients

32 patients with diagnosis of CIDP and fulfillment of neurophysiologic criteria for multifocal demyelinating polyradiculoneuropathy were randomized. Patients were excluded if they fulfilled criteria for multifocal motor neuropathy with conduction block, had systemic diseases that might cause neuropathy, had received treatment with steroids, IVIg, PE, or any immunosuppressant drug (aside from azathioprine) during the 6 weeks prior to randomization or had previous failure to respond to either IVIg or prednisolone.

Interventions

Patients were randomized to receive prednisolone followed by IVIg or IVIg followed by prednisolone. Prednisolone was delivered as an oral taper dosed once daily in the morning: 60 mg for 2 weeks, then 1 week each of 40 mg, 30 mg, 20 mg, 10 mg. IVIg infusions were given as 1.0 g/kg on 2 consecutive days or 2.0 g/kg in 24 hours. Each center was blinded to treatment allocation. Each patient received both an infusion and pill for the duration of each treatment period.

Outcomes

Primary outcome was the difference in a novel disability scale after 2 weeks. Secondary outcomes were changes in 10-m walk time and nine-hole pegboard time after 2 weeks and an assessment of each measure taking into account all time points.

KEY RESULTS

- Both treatments produced significant improvements in the primary outcome measure.
- There were slight but not significantly greater improvements favoring IVIg in both primary and secondary outcome measures.
- 32 patients completed the first treatment period, but 8 patients were withdrawn before reaching the 2-week outcome measure in the second treatment period. Six of these eight had received IVIg first.
- A serious adverse event (psychosis) attributable to treatment occurred in one patient while on prednisolone and none on IVIg.

STUDY CONCLUSIONS

The results of this trial confirm the efficacy of both oral steroids and IVIg in CIDP consistent with evidence from prior trials. There may be slightly more short-term efficacy with IVIg than with steroids.

COMMENTARY

This study compared prednisolone and IVIg for treatment of CIDP and again confirmed they are both efficacious but did not demonstrate clear superiority of one agent. The study was underpowered because of logistic constraints that shortened the enrollment period; additionally, eight patients were withdrawn from the study prior to its completion. Given the trend toward greater improvement with IVIg, it is possible a larger study with higher completion rate may demonstrate a significant difference. Notably, this study focused on immediate benefit of therapy and did not examine the benefit/burden of chronic therapy. In the intervening years since the 2001 publication of this study, these three agents remain first-line treatment with initial choice of agent dictated largely by disease severity, concurrent illness, venous access, treatment side effects, availability, and cost.

Question

Is IVIg superior to oral prednisolone in treatment of CIDP?

Answer

No, this study failed to demonstrate significant superiority of IVIg.

GLUCOCORTICOID STEROIDS FOR DUCHENNE MUSCULAR DYSTROPHY

CHAPTER 59

Randomized, Double-Blind Six-Month Trial of Prednisone in Duchenne's Muscular Dystrophy

Mendell JR, Moxley RT, Griggs RC, et al. *NEJM*. 1989;320(24):1592–1597

BACKGROUND

Duchenne's muscular dystrophy (DMD) is an X-linked recessive disorder caused by mutations in the dystrophin gene and results in progressive disability and death in early adulthood. At the time of this study, there were no treatments proven to improve or slow the disorder, and prior studies assessing prednisone in DMD demonstrated unclear benefit.

OBJECTIVES

To clarify the effect of prednisone in treatment of DMD.

METHODS

Randomized, placebo-controlled, double-blind trial over 6 months in the late 1980s at four neuromuscular centers in the United States.

Patients

103 patients 5 to 15 years of age who had DMD based on previously established clinical, laboratory, and diagnostic (but not genetic) testing were randomized to one of three intervention groups. There were no significant differences between the three groups in any baseline characteristics including age and functional/strength assessments.

Interventions

Three groups received one of the following daily oral treatments: placebo ($n = 36$), 0.75 mg/kg prednisone ($n = 33$), 1.5 mg/kg prednisone ($n = 34$). Participants and investigators were blinded to treatment assignments. Identification of patients taking prednisone may have been possible based on observable side effects such as Cushingoid appearance, but to minimize this bias clinical evaluations for strength/functional assessments and side effect screening were carried out by different individuals.

Outcomes

Average muscle strength was the primary outcome measurement of treatment efficacy. Secondary outcomes included contracture severity, timed functional testing, functional grade, ability to lift weights, and pulmonary function tests.

KEY RESULTS

- Both prednisone groups had significant improvement in average muscle strength as compared to placebo when tested at 1, 2, and 3 months, with a sustained effect at 6 months of treatment.

- Prednisone-treated groups improved significantly on the following secondary outcome measures as compared to placebo: timed functional testing, pulmonary function tests, ability to lift a kilogram weight, leg function grades.
- Prednisone-treated groups had significantly more urinary creatinine excretion than placebo group.
- Weight gain, Cushingoid appearance, and excessive hair growth were significantly greater in both prednisone groups than in the placebo group

STUDY CONCLUSIONS

A single daily dose of prednisone in an amount of 0.75 or 1.5 mg/kg administered for 6 months significantly improved muscle strength, pulmonary function, the ability to climb stairs, the time to rise from the floor, and the time to travel 9 m in patients with DMD. There was also an increase in urinary creatinine excretion, suggesting that an increase in muscle mass accompanied the increase in muscle strength.

COMMENTARY

This study demonstrated short-term benefit of steroids in muscle strength and functional ability in patients with DMD. Measurement of muscle strength is subject to poor interrater reliability, and assessments in this study may have been biased by the Cushingoid appearance of some subjects. However, significant improvement was also documented in the more objective secondary outcome measures. This study paved the way for additional studies, which also confirmed findings of improved strength, delay in cardiomyopathy, and delay in time to wheelchair dependence with prednisone. Based on the results of this and subsequent studies, the American Academy of Neurology now recommends prednisone (0.75 mg/kg/day or 10 mg/kg/week given over 2 weekend days) should be offered as treatment for boys with DMD who are 5 years of age or older. Benefits and side effects of steroid therapy are to be monitored, with side effects potentially limiting duration of treatment.

Question

Are oral steroids beneficial in the treatment of DMD?

Answer

Yes, oral steroids improve short-term muscle strength and functional ability in patients with DMD.

CHAPTER 60

RILUZOLE IN AMYOTROPHIC LATERAL SCLEROSIS

A Controlled Trial of Riluzole in Amyotrophic Lateral Sclerosis

Bensimon G, Lacomblez L, Meininger V. *NEJM*. 1994;330(9):585–591

BACKGROUND

Amyotrophic lateral sclerosis (ALS) is a progressive and fatal motor neuron disease with unknown cause. Some research suggests glutamate—the primary excitatory neurotransmitter in the CNS—may be involved in the pathogenesis. At the time of this study, there was no treatment known to influence survival.

OBJECTIVES

To evaluate the efficacy and safety of the antiglutamate agent riluzole in patients with ALS.

METHODS

Prospective, randomized, double-blind, placebo-controlled trial at seven centers in France between 1990 and 1992.

Patients

155 patients with probable or definite ALS (32 with bulbar-onset disease and 123 with limb-onset disease, 5 with familial ALS). Patients were excluded if objective testing had revealed any signs inconsistent with a diagnosis of ALS (e.g., paraproteinemia, focal lesions).

Interventions

Patients were randomized to receive 50 mg riluzole or tablets of identical-appearing placebo—both taken orally twice daily. Patient randomization was stratified by center of treatment and site of onset of disease (limb or bulbar). Patients and investigators were both blinded.

Outcomes

Primary efficacy outcomes were survival and functional status. Survival was determined by absence of death from any cause or tracheostomy. Secondary outcomes included muscle testing scores, measures of respiratory function, scores on the Clinical Global Impression of Change scale, and the patient's subjective evaluations of fasciculations, cramps, stiffness, and tiredness.

KEY RESULTS

- At 1 year, there was a statistically significant difference in survival: 74% of patients (57 of 77) in the riluzole group were still alive as compared with 58% (45 of 78) in the placebo group.

- Subgroup analysis indicates that the treatment effect was greater in patients with bulbar-onset disease than in those with limb-onset disease. For patients with bulbar-onset disease, 1 year survival rates were statistically significant between treatment groups: 73% (11 of 15) with riluzole and 35% (6 of 17) with placebo. For those with limb-onset disease, 1-year survival with riluzole vs. placebo was 74% and 64%, respectively ($p = 0.17$).
- After adjustment by age, duration of disease, forced vital capacity, bulbar function score, the tiredness score, and the stiffness score, the difference in survival between treatments was significant only at 12 months and not at the end of the placebo-controlled period (21 months).
- Adverse reactions to riluzole included asthenia, spasticity, mild elevations in aminotransferase levels.

STUDY CONCLUSIONS

Riluzole appears to slow the progression of ALS; it may improve survival in patients with disease of bulbar onset.

COMMENTARY

This study found modest improvement in survival for those treated with the antiglutamate agent riluzole but further post hoc analyses revealed this benefit extended only to those with bulbar-onset disease, a result for which the study was not adequately powered to assess. Moreover, when 24 patients included in the study who did not meet the a priori exclusion criteria are removed from statistical analysis, the effect of riluzole on mortality no longer achieves statistical significance. To date, the pathogenesis of ALS remains unknown and riluzole is the only treatment available aside from BiPAP, which has been shown to prolong survival as well.[1] Since the publication of this study riluzole at a dose of 50 mg twice daily is routinely offered to patients with ALS. Its modest benefit is estimated to result in an approximate 10% slowing of disease progression, but the benefit is nearly imperceptible to the patient—as demonstrated by absence of improvement in any patient-reported functional outcomes in this study. Riluzole is extremely expensive and whether its benefits exceed its cost remains a difficult but necessary conversation to have with each individual patient.

Question

Does riluzole prolong survival in ALS?

Answer

Unclear, it may improve survival in patients with bulbar-onset disease.

Reference

1. Kleopa KA, Sherman M, Neal B, et al. BiPAP improves survival and rate of pulmonary function decline in patients with ALS. *J Neurol Sci.* 1999;164(1):82–88.

CHAPTER 61

THYMECTOMY IN MYASTHENIA GRAVIS

Ayush Batra ■ Kate Brizzi ■ Joel Salinas ■ Nancy Wang

Randomized Trial of Thymectomy in Myasthenia Gravis

Wolfe GI, Kaminski HJ, Aban IB, et al. *NEJM*. 2016;375(6):511–522

BACKGROUND

MG is an autoimmune disease affecting the function of the neuromuscular junction. The thymus is suspected to have a role in disease pathogenesis, and thymectomy has historically been recommended in patients with known thymoma in the presence of disease. Prior to this trial, the role of thymectomy in nonthymomatous MG was unknown.

OBJECTIVES

To compare extended transsternal thymectomy plus alternate-day prednisone with alternate-day prednisone alone.

METHODS

Single-blind, multicenter, RCT from 2006 to 2012.

Patients

Patients aged 18 to 65 years with generalized nonthymomatous MG and disease duration less than 5 years; serum acetylcholine receptor antibody level of more than 1.0 nmol/L; and Myasthenia Gravis Foundation of America Clinical Classification scales II to IV. Exclusion criteria included thymoma; immunotherapy other than prednisone; previous thymectomy; pregnancy; and substantial medical illness.

Interventions

Participants were randomized to undergo thymectomy plus prednisone or prednisone alone. Prednisone was tapered according to patient symptom severity along a scaled protocol. Surveillance laboratory testing for complete blood count (CBC), glucose, hemoglobin A1c, and potassium was performed monthly and then quarterly.

Outcomes

Dual primary outcome of (1) time-weighted average quantitative MG score and (2) prednisone requirement over a 3-year period. Secondary outcomes included adverse events, quality of life self-report score, and rate of need for immunosuppression with azathioprine.

KEY RESULTS

- Thymectomy was associated with significantly lower time-weighted average quantitative MG score.
- Patients in the intervention group had significantly lower average requirement for alternate-day prednisone (44 vs. 60 mg).
- Fewer patients in the thymectomy group required immunosuppression with azathioprine (17% vs. 48%).
- Fewer hospitalizations for exacerbations in the thymectomy group.

STUDY CONCLUSIONS

Transsternal thymectomy in patients with nonthymomatous MG had improved dual primary outcomes over a 3-year period.

COMMENTARY

This study was the first to show the benefit of thymectomy in nonthymomatous MG. The results of this study show clinically meaningful reduction of symptoms related to the use of glucocorticoids and fewer hospitalizations related to MG exacerbations. The study was well designed in masking of the surgical intervention group and in its attempt to maximize generalizability of findings. Given a 3-year study duration, the long-term outcomes of the intervention remain unknown because differences between the groups may not remain significant over time. As a result of the study's findings, thymectomy may be offered to patients with MG even in the absence of thymoma. Future studies are needed to compare the use of novel immunosuppressive therapies to thymectomy.

Question

Does thymectomy in nonthymomatous MG improve clinical outcomes?

Answer

Yes, thymectomy in nonthymomatous MG improves patient symptoms and decreases need for additional immunosuppression.

SECTION 8

MOVEMENT DISORDERS

Todd Herrington ■ Abby L. Olsen

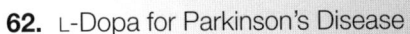

CHAPTER 62

L-DOPA FOR PARKINSON'S DISEASE

Efficacy of L-dopa in Treating Parkinsonism in 28 Patients

Cotzias GC, Papavasiliou PS, Gellene R. *NEJM*. 1969;280(7):337–345

BACKGROUND

The authors had previously demonstrated some efficacy of treating Parkinsonism with D,L-dopa, but this required large doses and had unfavorable toxicity, including granulocytopenia. The goal of this study was to demonstrate efficacy and a more favorable toxicity profile of the L-isomer.

OBJECTIVES

To demonstrate efficacy of L-dopa in a series of patients with Parkinsonism.

METHODS

Observational study of patients admitted to a metabolic ward.

Patients

28 patients with Parkinsonism who had an unsatisfactory response to conventional treatment.

Interventions

The intervention was L-dopa vs. lactose placebo. Patients received the placebo for 3 weeks, followed by 100 mg dopamine three times a day. The dose was then uptitrated as tolerated until an optimal dose was reached. There was extensive laboratory testing to monitor toxic effects.

Outcomes

Therapeutic effects (controlling Parkinsonism), side effects (CNS effects other than therapeutic ones), and toxicologic effects (those arising in peripheral organs) were assessed. A clinical scale was used to assess akinesia, rigidity, and tremor as the main aspects of Parkinsonism.

KEY RESULTS

- Every patient had at least partial improvement of some aspects of their Parkinsonism.
- Akinesia improved at the lowest doses, followed by rigidity and tremor.
- Improvement in performance was modest in 4 patients, moderate in 4, marked in 10, and dramatic in 10.
- Fluctuations in improvement throughout the day were seen in several patients.
- Side effects included nausea, vomiting, anorexia, mental effects, and involuntary movements.

STUDY CONCLUSIONS

L-Dopa leads to improvement in every aspect of Parkinsonism with a tolerable side effect profile when the dose is escalated slowly.

COMMENTARY

This landmark study, described in an accompanying editorial as "the most important contribution to medical therapy of a neurologic disease in the past 50 years," demonstrated that L-dopa was an effective therapy for Parkinsonism. Although the patient population in the study was heterogeneous, including a mixture of postencephalitic, vascular, and idiopathic Parkinson's disease, all patients had some degree of response. L-Dopa represented a significant therapeutic advance over D,L-dopa, requiring on average half the dose to achieve efficacy, resulting in improved toxicity and a higher proportion of improved patients. Large doses (3 g) were still required to achieve efficacy, and peripheral side effects emerged before neurologic improvement did. This observation paved the way for future studies on the addition of carbidopa to levodopa. Even today, this remains the most commonly used medication to treat Parkinson's disease.

Question

Is L-dopa effective in amelioration of Parkinsonism?

Answer

Yes, L-dopa improves tremor, rigidity, and akinesia with effects ranging from modest to dramatic and with a tolerable side effect profile.

CHAPTER 63

DEEP BRAIN STIMULATION FOR PARKINSON'S DISEASE

A Randomized Trial of Deep Brain Stimulation for Parkinson's Disease

Deuschl G, Schade-Brittinger C, Krack P, et al. *NEJM*. 2006;355(9):896–908

BACKGROUND

Although medical therapy is typically very effective in treating Parkinson's disease, with the progression of the disease patients exhibit fluctuations in their symptoms that are difficult to manage with medication alone. When this study was published, deep brain stimulation (DBS) of the subthalamic nucleus had been shown to improve symptoms in advanced Parkinson's disease in open studies, with symptom improvement of up to 5 years. This study was the first RCT comparing neurostimulation with best MM.

OBJECTIVES

To assess the effect of DBS of the subthalamic nucleus on quality of life and motor symptoms in patients with severe Parkinson's disease.

METHODS

Randomized pairs nonblinded multicenter trial.

Patients

156 patients with advanced Parkinson's disease and severe motor symptoms. All had disease for at least 5 years and were under age 75, with an average age of 60. Patients with dementia were excluded. Patients were enrolled in pairs and randomized after 6 weeks.

Interventions

DBS of the subthalamic nucleus combined with MM vs. MM alone. Surgery was performed on the bilateral subthalamic nucleus under local anesthesia.

Outcomes

Primary outcomes included changes from baseline to 6 months in quality of life, assessed by the Parkinson's Disease Questionnaire (PDQ-39), and severity of symptoms off medication for 12 hours, assessed with the Unified Parkinson's Disease Rating Scale, part III (UPDRS-III). Secondary outcomes included dyskinesia ratings, assessments of activities of daily living, cognitive and depression rating scales, and patient-reported hours of mobility.

KEY RESULTS

- Neurostimulation plus MM compared to MM alone led to significant improvement in both quality of life and motor symptoms at 6 months.
- Of 78 pairs of patients, in 50 pairs the patient treated with neurostimulation had greater improvement in quality of life, and in 55 pairs the patient had greater improvement in motor symptoms.
- Improvement in quality of life from baseline to 6 months was approximately 25% in the neurostimulation group, with no improvement in the medication group.
- Improvement in motor symptoms off medication was approximately 41% in the neurostimulation group, with no improvement in the medical therapy group.
- Total adverse events were more common in the medication group, but serious adverse events were more common in the neurostimulation group, including one fatal intracerebral hemorrhage.

STUDY CONCLUSIONS

Neurostimulation of the subthalamic nucleus combined with MM is more effective than MM alone in reducing severe motor symptoms and increasing quality of life at 6 months in patients with Parkinson's disease.

COMMENTARY

This is an important study and the first randomized trial of DBS for Parkinson's disease. Importantly, the study assessed motor symptoms off medication for 12 hours, highlighting the benefit of DBS, particularly in alleviating "off" symptoms. Subjects were able to reclaim approximately 5 hours/day, representing a significant improvement in functioning. The study is not without limitations, however. It is not blinded, and there is no sham surgery or placebo stimulation. Patients were followed for only 6 months, leaving the question of more long-term benefit of neurostimulation unanswered, although subsequent studies have shown that benefit is sustained at >5 years. Finally, there were serious adverse events in the neurostimulation group, including a fatal hemorrhage and a suicide.

Question

Does neurostimulation of the subthalamic nucleus improve quality of life and motor symptoms in patients with Parkinson's disease?

Answer

Yes, patients who received neurostimulation and medical therapy had significant improvement in both quality of life and motor symptoms at 6 months.

CHAPTER 64

DEEP BRAIN STIMULATION FOR DYSTONIA

Bilateral Deep Brain Stimulation of the Globus Pallidus in Primary Generalized Dystonia

Vidaihet M, Vercueil L, Houeto JL, et al. *NEJM.* 2005;352:459–467

BACKGROUND

Primary generalized dystonia causes severe disability and responds poorly to medical therapy. At the time of this publication, DBS of the globus pallidus had been shown to be efficacious in children, but there were limited data for adults, with only heterogeneous nonblinded small studies available. This study sought to assess the efficacy of DBS for primary generalized dystonia in a more controlled and standardized fashion.

OBJECTIVES

To assess the efficacy of DBS of the globus pallidus for primary generalized dystonia.

METHODS

Prospective controlled double-blind multicenter study.

Patients

22 patients with primary generalized dystonia who had severe impairment in activities of daily living. 7 patients had the torsin gene (DYT1) mutation. Inclusion criteria were clinical diagnosis of primary generalized dystonia, otherwise normal neurologic exam, normal MRI, absence of psychiatric disease, normal cognitive function, and severe impairment in the ability to perform activities of daily living despite MM.

Interventions

Patients were evaluated before surgery and at 3, 6, and 12 months postoperatively during neurostimulation after having received bilateral leads implanted in the globus pallidus.

Outcomes

The movement and disability subscores of the Burke–Fahn–Marsden Dystonia Scale were used as primary outcomes at 12 months. Movement scores were measured by videotaped sessions performed by a blinded observer. Scores were also assessed at 3 months in a double-blind evaluation in the presence and absence of neurostimulation on separate days. Other secondary outcomes included quality of life, cognition, and mood, assessed at baseline and 12 months using the Medical Outcomes Study (MOS) 36-Item Short-Form General Health Survey, the MMSE, and the Beck Depression Inventory, respectively.

KEY RESULTS

- Movement scores improved significantly between baseline and 12 months in patients undergoing neurostimulation.
- The patients with the most improvement in movement had diffuse hyperkinetic involuntary movements prior to DBS, whereas four patients with either little improvement or worsening movements had severe tonic abnormal postures prior to DBS.
- Disability score improved significantly at every time point, and general health and physical functioning were significantly improved at 12 months.
- Improvement was not correlated with sex, age, duration of disease, DYT1 status, or scores on the Burke–Fahn–Marsden Dystonia Scale.
- There were five adverse events in three patients. All resolved without permanent sequelae.

STUDY CONCLUSIONS

DBS of the globus pallidus for primary generalized dystonia was both safe and effective.

COMMENTARY

Although there were numerous case reports demonstrating benefits of DBS for dystonia, this study is the first controlled double-blinded multicenter trial to demonstrate clearly that DBS of the bilateral internal globus pallidus is an effective and safe treatment for primary generalized dystonia. Benefit was both early (3 months) and sustained (12 months). Among patients who improved, there was benefit in the neck, trunk, and limbs, but not in facial movement or speech. Additionally, the four patients who failed to improve had severe tonic posturing, whereas those that improved the most had phasic movements. These observations might influence clinical decision-making when selecting patients for surgery in the future. The study was limited by its small size (22 patients) and preponderance of pediatric patients (17/22 were under 18), which may limit its applicability to adult-onset dystonia.

Question

Is DBS of the globus pallidus an effective therapy for primary generalized dystonia?

Answer

Yes, patients had sustained significantly improved movement and disability scores after receiving DBS of the bilateral internal globus pallidus.

CHAPTER 65

L-DOPA VS. MAO-B INHIBITORS IN PARKINSON'S DISEASE

Long-Term Effectiveness of Dopamine Agonists and Monoamine Oxidase B Inhibitors Compared with Levodopa as Initial Treatment for Parkinson's Disease: A Large, Open-Label, Pragmatic Randomized Trial

PD Med Collaborative Group, Gray R, Ives N, et al. *Lancet.* 2014;384(9949):1196–1205

BACKGROUND

Levodopa, dopamine agonists, and monoamine oxidase B inhibitors (MAOBIs) all have established efficacy for Parkinson's disease, but it is unclear which of these classes of medications provides the most effective long-term control of symptoms when used as initial treatment for Parkinson's disease. Earlier exposure to levodopa had been associated with the earlier development of dyskinesias, prompting some providers to defer starting levodopa in favor of dopamine agonists and MAOBIs. However, dopamine agonists are associated with nonmotor side effects and MAOBIs with higher mortality in some studies. The goal of this study was to determine which class of therapy provided the best relief of symptoms over time.

OBJECTIVES

To determine whether initial treatment with levodopa, dopamine agonists, or MAOBI results in better long-term control of symptoms.

METHODS

Open-label randomized multicenter trial from 2000 to 2009.

Patients

1,620 patients with newly diagnosed Parkinson's disease who were untreated or treated for <6 months.

Interventions

Patients were randomized between levodopa-sparing therapy (MAOBI or dopamine agonist) or levodopa alone. If symptoms were not controlled by the standard dose of an MAOBI or the maximum tolerated dose of a dopamine agonist, levodopa could be added.

Outcomes

The primary outcome was mobility score on the Parkinson's Disease Questionnaire (PDQ-39) quality of life assessment. There were numerous secondary outcomes, including PDQ-39 subscores, cognition, compliance, dyskinesias and motor fluctuations, admissions to hospital or institution, mortality, and quality-adjusted life-years (QALYs). Outcomes were measured at baseline, 6 months, 1 year, and annually thereafter. Median follow-up was 3 years.

KEY RESULTS

- Mobility scores were statistically significantly better in patients who received levodopa compared to those who received a levodopa-sparing agent, although the magnitude of the difference was small and fell below the predetermined threshold of clinical significance.
- Rates of dementia, admissions to institutions, and death were not significantly different among treatment groups.
- More patients discontinued MAOBI and dopamine agonists due to side effects compared to those who discontinued levodopa.
- Early initiation of levodopa was associated with earlier development of dyskinesias. However, rates of dyskinesias had equalized between groups by 7 years.

STUDY CONCLUSIONS

Treating with levodopa as opposed to a levodopa-sparing agent results in very small but persistent benefits in patient-related mobility scores, with a more favorable side effect profile.

COMMENTARY

The most important aspect of this study is not that it demonstrated a statistically significant benefit of levodopa over levodopa-sparing agents as initial treatment for Parkinson's disease. Rather, this study is important in allaying some fears regarding the popular idea that patients should be treated with a dopamine-sparing agent to improve the long-term efficacy of levodopa and to delay development of levodopa-related side effects. The authors show that levodopa efficacy was maintained, with a more favorable side effect profile, although there was earlier development of dyskinesias in the levodopa group. Potential limitations to the study include the somewhat heterogeneous population (e.g., 5% of patients with a Parkinson-plus syndrome rather than idiopathic Parkinson's disease) and the heterogeneous medication use and dosing within a particular class of medication. In addition, a few patients in the study were very young (<60 years old), and those patients may be at the most risk of developing levodopa-related dyskinesias, so it remains debatable whether these patients might benefit from a levodopa-sparing agent early in treatment.

Question

For early Parkinson's disease, is there any benefit to starting levodopa over levodopa-sparing agents?

Answer

Yes, levodopa is statistically but not clinically superior to levodopa-sparing agents in terms of quality of life, but at the risk of earlier dyskinesias.

CHAPTER 66

PROPRANOLOL TREATMENT FOR ESSENTIAL TREMOR

Efficacy of Chronic Propranolol Therapy in Action Tremors of the Familial, Senile, or Essential Varieties

Winkler GF, Young RR. *NEJM*. 1974;290(18):984–988

BACKGROUND

Action tremor can be disabling to patients, causing social embarrassment and impairment in activities of daily living. At the time when this paper was published, there were no nonsedating, nonaddictive treatments for action tremor. The first author of this study reportedly noticed that a patient receiving propranolol for paroxysmal atrial tachycardia had marked improvement of her tremor, which motivated the study.

OBJECTIVES

To determine the efficacy of propranolol for action tremor.

METHODS

Double-blind placebo-controlled crossover study

Patients

24 patients with severe action tremor (described as 14 with familial tremor, 2 with senile tremor, 8 with essential tremor), age 31 to 79, with symptoms ranging from 1 to 60 years.

Interventions

Propranolol (at a dose of 60 to 160 mg/day in 3 to 4 divided doses) was compared to placebo. After 2 weeks of either propranolol or placebo, patients switched to the other arm of the study. If there was no difference noted between propranolol vs. placebo during the first trial, the trial was repeated with double the dose.

Outcomes

Patients assessed their tremor severity subjectively. Clinicians then assessed the amplitude of tremor on a four-point scale for each limb in various postures and while holding a full cup. Handwriting specimens were obtained. Accelerometers were used to measure frequency and amplitude.

KEY RESULTS

- Most subjects experienced dramatic relief of tremor within 24 to 48 hours of starting propranolol, and this improvement disappeared within the same time period after stopping propranolol.
- 20 of 24 patients reported subjective improvement with propranolol; no one reported subjective improvement on placebo.
- A similar number of patients improved when scored by examiners.
- Tremor amplitude but not frequency was significantly reduced by propranolol.
- Handwriting improved in 15 of 18 patients whose tremor degraded handwriting at baseline.

STUDY CONCLUSIONS

Propranolol is an effective treatment for the majority of patients with action tremor.

COMMENTARY

This is the first demonstration that a nonsedating, nonaddictive medication can alleviate the symptoms of action tremor. As the most common movement disorder, the availability of an effective, safe treatment for action tremor has been beneficial for affected individuals. The authors raise the interesting point that propranolol is not effective for other types of tremor, including cerebellar and resting tremors, making the diagnosis of tremor subtype more clinically important than before.

Question

Is propranolol effective for action tremor?

Answer

Yes, propranolol is an effective and safe medication for action tremor.

CHAPTER 67

RASAGILINE IN PARKINSON'S DISEASE

A Double-Blind, Delayed-Start Trial of Rasagiline in Parkinson's Disease

Olanow CW, Rascol O, Hauser R, et al. *NEJM*. 2009;361(13):1268–1278

BACKGROUND

At the time of this publication, there were established therapies for treating the symptoms of Parkinson's disease, including the monoamine oxidase type B (MAO-B) inhibitors such as rasagiline and selegiline. There were no established disease-modifying therapies, however. The authors used a delayed-start trial to assess whether rasagiline has a disease-modifying effect, reasoning that if persistent differences are seen between patients who received the drug early and those who received it late, this cannot be explained by control of symptoms alone because everyone is eventually receiving the drug.

OBJECTIVES

To determine whether rasagiline has a disease-modifying effect on Parkinson's disease.

METHODS

Double-blind, placebo-controlled, multicenter delayed-start RCT.

Patients

1,176 patients with untreated Parkinson's disease. Patients were men and women 30 to 80 yearsof age. Patients who had previously received any anti-Parkinsonian medication for more than 3 weeks or who had received an MAO-B inhibitor within the previous 120 days were excluded. Patients with severe Parkinson's or atypical or secondary Parkinsonism were excluded. Mean duration of disease was 4.5 months.

Interventions

Patients were randomized to receive 1 or 2 mg rasagiline for 72 weeks, or placebo for 36 weeks, followed by rasagiline. They were not permitted to receive any additional Parkinson's medication. Patients were assessed at baseline and at 4, 12, 24, 36, 42, 48, 54, 60, 66, and 72 weeks.

Outcomes

Outcomes were based on the Unified Parkinson's Disease Rating Scale (UPDRS). There were three outcomes: superiority to placebo in the rate of change in the UPDRS score between weeks 12 and 36, superiority to delayed-start treatment in the change in the score between baseline and week 72, and noninferiority to delayed-start treatment in the rate of change in the score between weeks 48 and 72.

KEY RESULTS

- Rasagiline at either dose had beneficial effects on symptoms.
- Patients who received the 1-mg dose met all three outcomes.
- Patients who received the 2-mg dose met two of the three outcomes: a smaller increase in the UPDRS from week 12 to 36, and noninferiority compared to the delayed-start group.
- In post hoc analysis of patients with the highest quartile initial UPDRS score, the 2-mg dose did provide a statistically significant benefit from baseline to 72 weeks.
- If only patients with the lowest three quartiles of UPDRS scores at baseline were included, neither dose met all three prior end points.

STUDY CONCLUSIONS

At the 1-mg dose, rasagiline lessened the degree of worsening of the UPDRS from 12 to 36 weeks, and this benefit persisted at the 72-week time point, suggesting a possible slowing of disease progression beyond symptomatic improvement. This finding was not replicated at the 2-mg dose.

COMMENTARY

This study highlights the difficulty of assessing potential disease-modifying effects of medications that have symptomatic benefits when patient symptoms are the only metric of disease progression (i.e., in the absence of a suitable biomarker). This study suggested that rasagiline might slow the progression of Parkinson's disease. The results were inconclusive because the three primary end points were met by the 1-mg but not the 2-mg dose. One possible confounder was that patients in the study had very early disease, and post hoc analysis suggested that patients with more advanced disease at presentation might benefit the most from rasagiline, although the sample size was small. Another possibility is that the 2-mg dose was actually too high; evidence from preclinical studies supports that lower doses act through neurotropic factors and are neuroprotective, an effect that could be lost at higher doses. The possible neuroprotective benefit from treatment with rasagiline remains controversial, and further study is needed.

Question

Is rasagiline an effective disease-modifying therapy for Parkinson's disease?

Answer

Maybe, rasagiline at doses of 1 mg/day demonstrated benefits suggestive of a disease-modifying effect, but this remains controversial.

CHAPTER 68

BOTULINUM A TOXIN FOR DYSTONIA

Botulinum A Toxin for Cranial-Cervical Dystonia: A Double-Blind Placebo-Controlled Study

Jankovic J, Orman J. *Neurology*. 1987;37(4):616–623

BACKGROUND

At the time of this publication, open-label studies had demonstrated utility for botulinum toxin A in treatment of strabismus, blepharospasm, hemifacial spasm, and focal dystonias, but no randomized trials had been performed.

OBJECTIVES

To determine the efficacy of botulinum toxin A as a treatment for dystonia.

METHODS

Double-blind, placebo-controlled, single-center trial.

Patients

22 patients were enrolled in the randomized trial: 10 with blepharospasm and 12 with oromandibular-cervical dystonia. All patients were disabled despite pharmacologic or surgical therapy. There was a preliminary open-label study with nine patients to determine the range of effective dosages and adverse reactions and to allow investigators to gain experience with the injection technique. Two of these nine patients were subsequently randomized into the main trial.

Interventions

Electromyography (EMG) was used to localize the cervical muscles with the maximal involuntary contraction to be targeted for injection. The starting dose was 25 units per injection site except for patients with pharyngeal and laryngeal dystonias. If the initial dose was ineffective, the injection was repeated 1 month later using a double dose. If the second injection was ineffective, the patient was crossed over to the alternate treatment.

Outcomes

Patients were interviewed 1 week after injection and then monthly. The severity of blepharospasm and oromandibular dystonia was assessed by their neurologist with the 0 to 4 Fahn Rating Scale. Other forms of dystonia were assessed with the Hyperkinesia Rating Scale. Patients also kept a daily diary and rated their disability on the Fahn–Marsden Dystonia Scale. Patients were videotaped at each appointment and rated by other blinded neurologists.

KEY RESULTS

- Seven of nine patients in the open-label trial improved after the first injection. All nine improved after the second. The peak effect was at 2.5 weeks and the mean duration was 6.3 weeks.
- No blepharospasm patients improved in the placebo arm of the controlled trial, and all patients improved in the botulinum toxin arm. There was 71.6% improvement in the dystonia severity rating score, 60.7% improvement in the self-assessment score, and 38.9% improvement on the videotape score. The peak effect was 3.7 weeks and the duration was 12.5 weeks.
- For the oromandibular dystonia patients, more improved with the toxin than with placebo, but the difference was not statistically significant.

STUDY CONCLUSIONS

Blepharospasm patients treated with botulinum toxin A had significant improvement as rated by dystonia severity rating score, dystonia self-assessment score, and a blinded videotape score. Although oromandibular dystonia patients improved in the open-label arm of the trial, the difference between botulinum toxin A and placebo was not statistically significant in the controlled arm.

COMMENTARY

This was the first randomized controlled trial to demonstrate efficacy for botulinum toxin A in the treatment of dystonia. There are some limitations to the study, including its small size and the fact that it is an operator-dependent technique (requiring familiarity with EMG as performed here), raising issues of generalizability to other centers. Although significant benefit was demonstrated only for blepharospasm and not for other dystonias, this study paved the way for additional trials looking at higher doses of botulinum toxin A, which have now become the standard of care. The therapy was well tolerated with only transient local side effects.

Question

Is botulinum toxin A an efficacious treatment for focal dystonias?

Answer

Yes, botulinum toxin A is effective in treatment for blepharospasm.

James Stankiewicz ■ Tamara B. Kaplan

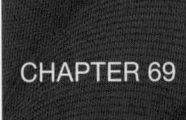

| CHAPTER 69 | PROGRESSIVE MULTIFOCAL LEUKOENCEPHALOPATHY AFTER TREATMENT WITH NATALIZUMAB |

Evaluation of Patients Treated with Natalizumab for Progressive Multifocal Leukoencephalopathy

Yousry TA, Major EO, Ryschkewitsch C, et al. *NEJM*. 2006;354(9):924–933

BACKGROUND

Progressive multifocal leukoencephalopathy (PML) is a rare but serious infectious demyelinating brain disease that occurs most frequently in immunocompromised patients and has been reported in multiple sclerosis (MS) patients treated with the recombinant humanized antibody natalizumab. As a consequence of the reported PML cases, the drug was withdrawn from the market in 2005 after it was approved in 2004. At the time of this study, the true incidence of PML associated with natalizumab treatment was unknown.

OBJECTIVE

To determine whether PML had developed in any other patients treated with natalizumab and to better understand the overall incidence of PML associated with natalizumab treatment.

METHODS

Retrospective cohort study including patients who had participated in recent clinical trials of natalizumab from 2004 to 2005.

Patients

Overall, 3,116 patients were enrolled who had been exposed to natalizumab. This included 1,869 patients with MS and 1,247 patients with Crohn's disease (CD) or rheumatoid arthritis (RA).

Interventions

Local physicians were asked to evaluate each patient, including a detailed history, physical exam, and neurologic exam. They were also asked to arrange for brain MRI and obtain CSF. The information was reviewed locally, and any cases concerning for PML were forwarded to an Independent adjudication committee (IAC), and 44 were referred to the expert panel because of clinical findings of possible PML, abnormalities on MRI, or a high plasma load of JC Virus (JCV). No patient had detectable JCV DNA in CSF.

Outcomes

The primary outcome was confirmed cases of PML.

KEY RESULTS
- 2,046 patients with MS, 1,342 patients with RA or CD, and 2 patients with MS not in clinical trials were cleared for PML by the IAC.
- One patient with MS in a clinical study declined further follow-up.
- Zero cases of PML were confirmed by the IAC.
- PML was ruled out in 43 of the 44 patients, but could not be ruled out in one patient because CSF and follow-up MRI were not available.

STUDY CONCLUSIONS
No new PML cases were identified in this study, suggesting a risk of PML of roughly 1 in 1,000 patients treated with natalizumab for a mean of 17.9 months.

COMMENTARY

Prior to this study, there were several case reports of PML in patients who had received treatment with natalizumab, but the actual risk of PML was difficult to assess. This study spanned multiple clinical trials and was performed to help guide whether or not natalizumab could be safely administered. The authors do acknowledge several potential limitations to this study. This study does not answer questions about the duration of exposure to natalizumab needed to raise the risk of PML. The authors also note that all participants had discontinued natalizumab at the time of the study, and thus the study can only evaluate prior treatment. Based on this study, it was considered that the estimated risk of PML was acceptable given the considerable therapeutic benefits of natalizumab, and the drug was reintroduced in the market in June 2006 and approved by the FDA and European Medicines Agency for highly active relapsing-remitting MS. Currently, this medication is used as a highly effective treatment for relapsing-remitting MS. A serum JCV antibody test has been developed that can help further stratify risk.

Question

Does prior use of natalizumab confer risk for the development of PML?

Answer

Yes, the study determined that exposure to natalizumab conferred an overall risk of 1:1,000 for PML.

CHAPTER 70

GLUCOCORTICOIDS FOR OPTIC NEURITIS: THE OPTIC NEURITIS TREATMENT TRIAL

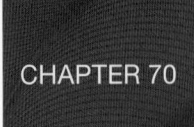

A Randomized, Controlled Trial of Corticosteroids in the Treatment of Acute Optic Neuritis

Beck RW, Cleary PA, Anderson MM, et al; The Optic Neuritis Study Group. *NEJM*. 1992;326(9):581–588

BACKGROUND

Optic neuritis is an inflammatory condition of the optic nerve characterized by unilateral visual loss that typically worsens over a few days and is often associated with MS. This was the first major study that provided information on the natural history of optic neuritis, the role of steroids in treatment, and the risk of developing MS.

OBJECTIVE

To assess the effects of corticosteroids on visual recovery of patients with acute optic neuritis.

METHODS

Randomized case-controlled study starting in 1988 with subsequent prospective cohort analysis.

Patients

The study enrolled 457 patients with acute optic neuritis. These patients were enrolled within 8 days of symptom onset with unilateral vision loss in an eye that had not had optic neuritis previously.

Interventions

Patients were randomly assigned to either oral prednisone (1 mg/kg/day) for 14 days with a 4-day taper; IV MP (250 mg QID for 3 days) followed by oral prednisone (1 mg/kg/day) for 11 days with a 4-day taper; or oral placebo for 14 days. Patients were randomized and received their allocated intervention within 8 days of symptom onset.

Outcomes

The primary visual outcomes were visual acuity and contrast sensitivity over a 6-month follow-up period.

> ## KEY RESULTS
> - Visual function recovered faster in the group that received IV MP compared to placebo.
> - The difference between the two groups decreased at 6 months, but the group that received IV MP had significantly better contrast sensitivity and color vision but

not better visual acuity ($p = 0.66$). A trend was seen toward better visual fields ($p = 0.054$).
- The rate of new optic neuritis in either eye was highest in the group that received oral prednisone.

STUDY CONCLUSIONS

IV MP followed by oral prednisone speeds the recovery of visual loss due to optic neuritis. Oral prednisone, as prescribed in this study, is ineffective and increases the risk of new episodes of optic neuritis.

COMMENTARY

This trial was the first large RCT to assess optic neuritis treatment. After the publication of this trial, there were several other extended follow-up periods. These data allowed authors to draw further conclusions about the risk of MS years after developing optic neuritis. Of note, a meta-analysis of three trials, including this one, that compared treatment with IV MP to placebo, found no benefit of treatment on visual outcomes at 6 months and at 1 year.[1] Also, in a subsequent follow-up study at 10 years, the risk of recurrent optic neuritis remained higher in the oral prednisone group when compared with the IV-treated group (44% vs. 29%), but there was no longer a significant difference between the oral prednisone and placebo groups.[2] A secondary objective of this study group at a later follow-up point was to investigate the relationship between optic neuritis and MS. Although the incidence rates for MS were 16.2% vs. 32.4% and 35.9% in patients with 2 or more white matter lesions on MRI, at 5 years, there were no differences in the rates of MS between treatment groups.[3]

Question

Do corticosteroids aid in the recovery of optic neuritis?

Answer

Yes. IV MP but not oral prednisone speeds the recovery of optic neuritis, but does not alter long-term outcome with regard to visual acuity.

References
1. Gal RL, Vedula SS, Beck R. Corticosteroids for treating optic neuritis. *Cochrane Database Syst Rev.* 2012;4:CD001430.
2. Beck RW, Gal RL, Bhatti MT, et al; Optic Neuritis Study Group. Visual function more than 10 years after optic neuritis: experience of the optic neuritis treatment trial. *Am J Ophthalmol.* 2004;137(1):77–83.
3. Optic Neuritis Study Group. The 5-year risk of MS after optic neuritis: experience of the optic neuritis treatment trial. *Neurology.* 1997;49(5):1404–1413.

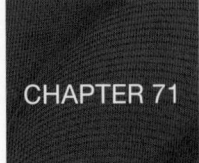

NEUROMYELITIS OPTICA ANTIBODY IN THE DIAGNOSIS OF NEUROMYELITIS OPTICA

CHAPTER 71

A Serum Autoantibody Marker of Neuromyelitis Optica: Distinction from Multiple Sclerosis

Lennon VA, Wingerchuk DM, Kryzer TJ, et al. *Lancet*. 2004;364(9451):2106–2112

BACKGROUND

Neuromyelitis optica (NMO) is an inflammatory demyelinating disease that affects the spinal cord and optic nerves. Historically, it was often misdiagnosed as MS; however, the two diseases differ in their natural history, pathophysiology, treatment, and prognosis. Until this publication, there were no unique biomarkers to distinguish the two diseases.

OBJECTIVES

To assess the capacity of NMO-IgG to distinguish NMO and related disorders from MS.

METHODS

Cross-sectional study of serum from patients with the appropriate clinical criteria from 1998 to 2003.

Patients

Serum was obtained and tested from 102 North American patients with clinically defined NMO or syndromes that suggested a high-risk NMO such as optic–spinal disease. In addition, 12 Japanese patients with optic–spinal MS were included. Control patients had MS, other myelopathies, optic neuropathies, and miscellaneous disorders. In addition, 14 patients were included who were incidentally shown to have NMO-IgG among 85,000 patients tested for suspected paraneoplastic autoimmune conditions.

Interventions

Serum samples were obtained from all study subjects and were tested by an indirect immunofluorescence assay, which identified a distinctive NMO-IgG staining pattern. Selected positive and negative serum samples were also tested on sections of mouse midbrain, spinal cord, and liver in order to localize the regions where the patients' IgG bound.

Outcomes

The primary outcome of this study was to establish the sensitivity and specificity for NMO-IgG in NMO.

KEY RESULTS

The sensitivity and specificity for NMO-IgG were 73% (95% CI = 60–86) and 91% (95% CI = 79–100) for NMO and 58% (95% CI = 30–86) and 100% (95% CI = 66–100) for those identified as optic–spinal MS (which is now considered to be the same as NMO).

- NMO-IgG was detected in half of patients with high-risk syndromes.
- Of 14 seropositive cases identified incidentally, 12 had NMO or a high-risk syndrome for the disease.
- In mice, NMO-IgG immunofluorescence was in a distribution suggestive of an antigen at the blood–brain barrier.

STUDY CONCLUSIONS

NMO-IgG is a specific autoantibody of NMO and binds at or near the blood–brain barrier. It distinguishes NMO from MS. Asian optic–spinal MS seems to be the same condition as NMO.

COMMENTARY

The authors described an IgG autoantibody (NMO-IgG) that is highly specific for NMO, and the presence of this specific serum autoantibody can differentiate NMO from MS. No biomarker had previously been described. Because of this discovery, NMO became the first inflammatory demyelinating disorder of the CNS to have a defined autoantigen. This discovery has enabled physicians to use a serologic test to help support the diagnosis of the disease and has helped to define an NMO spectrum of disorders. Further refinements in the quality of the assay have been made, further increasing the sensitivity and specificity. This study also paved the way for the discovery that NMO-IgG is actually directed against aquaporin-4 (AQP-4), a water channel that is highly expressed in optic nerves, spinal cord, and certain areas of the brain stem.

Question

Is NMO-IgG an appropriate biomarker to aid the diagnosis of NMO?

Answer

Yes, this autoantibody is highly specific for NMO and allows practitioners to distinguish between MS and NMO.

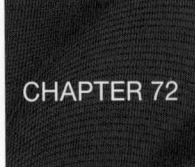

CORRELATION BETWEEN MRI FINDINGS AND DISABILITY IN MULTIPLE SCLEROSIS

CHAPTER 72

A Longitudinal Study of Abnormalities on MRI and Disability from Multiple Sclerosis
Brex PA, Ciccarelli O, O'Riordan JI, et al. *NEJM*. 2002;346:158–164

BACKGROUND
Prior to this study, it was well recognized that in patients who develop isolated syndromes suggestive of MS, such as optic neuritis or brainstem or spinal cord syndromes, the presence of T2-weighted lesions on MRI of the brain increases the likelihood of developing MS. However, the correlation between these T2 lesions and long-term disability was unknown prior to this prospective study.

OBJECTIVES
To determine the relation between early lesion volume, changes in volume, and long-term disability in patients with isolated syndromes that are clinically suggestive of MS.

METHODS
Prospective cohort study of patients presenting between 1984 and 1987.

Patients
71 patients in a serial MRI study of patients with isolated syndromes were reassessed after a mean of 14.1 years. Disability was measured with the use of Kurtzke's Expanded Disability Status Scale (EDSS; possible range, 0 to 10, with a higher score indicating a greater degree of disability).

Interventions
MRI data were available for assessments at base line and at 5, 10, and 14 years. Imaging was performed on a 0.5-T scanner at baseline and 5 years and on a 1.5-T scanner at 10 and 14 years.

Outcomes
Outcomes assessed include degree of disability and changes in MRI findings.

KEY RESULTS
- Clinically definite MS developed in 44 out of 50 patients (88%) with abnormal results on MRI at presentation and in 4 of 21 patients (19%) with normal results on MRI.
- The median EDSS score at follow-up for those with MS was 3.25 (range, 0 to 10); 31% had an EDSS score of 6 or more (including three patients whose deaths were due to MS).

- Patients with worse clinical outcomes had larger numbers and volumes of lesions on MRI at baseline and larger increases in lesion volume over time.
- The EDSS score at 14 years correlated moderately with lesion volume on MRI at 5 years ($r = 0.60$) and with the increase in lesion volume over the first 5 years ($r = 0.61$).

STUDY CONCLUSIONS
NA

COMMENTARY

This study showed that the EDSS score at 14 years correlated significantly with lesion volumes on MRI at all of the earlier time points, indicating that the lesion volume at any time contributes to the development of later disability. This study is an important natural history study. It is unlikely that a similar study could be done now given the wide array of disease modifying treatments (DMTs) which reduce MRI lesions over time. The study suggests that the number of lesions and the lesion volume on MRI in patients with early MS are moderately predictive of long-term disability. Given only moderate correlation, the authors point out that MRI lesion volume alone should not be used as the sole determinant when deciding about DMTs. However, this data help support the trend toward early use of DMT in patients with lesion accumulation/expansion, suggestive of MS. One important weaknesses of this study is the change in MRI technology over time. However, authors note that the degree of volume change seen in lesions was large enough to not be missed significantly on earlier scans. Overall, this study suggests that lesion volume on MRI is of prognostic value in assessing the risk of future disability.

Question

Does lesion volume on MRI predict long-term disability?

Answer

Yes, there is a moderate correlation between lesion volume on MRI and long-term disability as measured by EDSS.

CHAPTER 73

THE ASSOCIATION OF VITAMIN D LEVELS AND MULTIPLE SCLEROSIS

Serum 25-Hydroxyvitamin D Levels and Risk of Multiple Sclerosis

Munger KL, Levin LI, Hollis BW, et al. *JAMA*. 2006;296:2832–2838

BACKGROUND

The global distribution of MS increases with distance from the equator in both Northern and Southern hemispheres. A possible explanation for this interesting observation is that sunlight exposure and vitamin D levels also decrease with distance from the equator. Prior to this study, some epidemiologic and experimental evidence suggested that high levels of vitamin D may decrease the risk of MS. This was the first prospective study to address this hypothesis.

OBJECTIVES

To examine whether levels of 25-hydroxyvitamin D are associated with risk of MS.

METHODS

Prospective nested case-control study among more than 7 million US military personnel. Cases obtained were from databases from 1992 through 2004.

Patients

MS cases ($n = 257$) were identified through Army and Navy physical disability databases, and diagnoses were confirmed by medical record review. For each of the 257 cases, there were two controls that were matched by age, sex, race/ethnicity, and dates of blood collection.

Interventions

Vitamin D status was estimated by averaging 25-hydroxyvitamin D levels of two or more serum samples collected before the date of initial MS symptoms.

Outcomes

The main outcome measure included the odds ratios (ORs) of MS associated with continuous or categorical levels of serum 25-hydroxyvitamin D within each racial/ethnic group.

KEY RESULTS

- The risk of MS significantly decreased with increasing levels of 25-hydroxyvitamin D among whites (148 cases, 296 controls) with an OR of 0.59 (95% CI = 0.36–0.97) for a 50-nmol/L increase in 25-hydroxyvitamin D.
- Individuals were also classified under five predefined categories of 25-hydroxyvitamin D by 25-nmol/L increments. In the categorical analyses, the ORs for each category showed significance ($p = 0.02$) across quintiles.

- There was a strong inverse relationship with MS risk and 25-hydroxyvitamin D levels measured before age 20 years.
- There was no significant association between vitamin D and MS risk among blacks and Hispanics (109 cases, 218 controls), who had lower 25-hydroxyvitamin D levels than whites.

STUDY CONCLUSIONS

The results suggest that high circulating levels of vitamin D are associated with a lower risk of MS.

COMMENTARY

One potential environmental risk factor thought to be involved in increased susceptibility to MS is reduced levels of vitamin D. This large prospective study found that the risk of MS decreased with increasing serum levels of 25-hydroxyvitamin D. However, this association was not seen with blacks and Hispanics, but the authors suggest this could be because of the smaller sample size of this population. This study does not prove that decreased vitamin D levels actually causes MS. Rather, it suggests that high levels of vitamin D in the serum are associated with a lower risk of MS. Subsequent studies have confirmed this finding and extended it by revealing that patients diagnosed with MS who have higher vitamin D levels show less disease activity by relapses and MRI. Whether vitamin D supplementation may alter possibility or developing MS or may help attenuate disease after a diagnosis of MS requires further study.

Question

Are high circulating levels of vitamin D associated with a lower risk of developing MS?

Answer

Yes, the risk of MS significantly decreases with increasing levels of 25-hydroxyvitamin D, specifically among white patients.

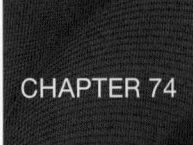

RATE OF PREGNANCY-RELATED RELAPSE IN MULTIPLE SCLEROSIS

CHAPTER 74

Rate of Pregnancy-Related Relapse in Multiple Sclerosis
Confavreux C, Hutchinson M, Hours MM, et al. *NEJM*. 1998;339(5):285–291

BACKGROUND
MS affects women of childbearing age. Prior to this study, it was suspected that there was a decreased rate of relapse during pregnancy and an increase in the postpartum period; however, these prior studies were small and some had reached different conclusions. This was the first large-scale prospective study to assess the effects of pregnancy on the natural history of MS.

OBJECTIVES
This study aimed to investigate the natural history of MS in pregnant women. Specifically, the study was designed to determine the effect of pregnancy and the postpartum state on the course of the disease, along with that of breast-feeding and epidural analgesia.

METHODS
Multicenter, prospective, observational study with recruitment from 1993 through 1995.

Patients
254 women (246 with relapsing MS) and 269 pregnancies. Each patient's first pregnancy leading to a live birth was included for analysis, for a total of 227 pregnancies.

Interventions
Patients were followed for at least 12 months postpartum. Women were followed during their pregnancies and for up to 12 months after delivery to determine the rate of relapse per trimester and the score on the Kurtzke Expanded Disability Status Scale (EDSS) (range 0 to 10, with higher scores indicating more severe disability).

Outcomes
Outcomes measured included degree of disability and rate of relapse.

KEY RESULTS
- The mean ($\pm$SD) rate of relapse was 0.7 ± 0.9 per woman per year in the year before pregnancy, it was 0.5 ± 1.3 during the first trimester ($p = 0.03$ for the comparison with the rate before pregnancy), 0.6 ± 1.6 during the second trimester ($p = 0.17$), and 0.2 ± 1.0 during the third trimester ($p < 0.001$).
- The rate significantly increased to 1.2 ± 2.0 during the first 3 months postpartum and then returned to the prepregnancy rate.

- Overall, compared to prepregnancy, annualized relapse rate fell by 70% during the third trimester.
- Neither epidural analgesia nor breast-feeding increased the risk of relapse or of worsening disability in the postpartum period. However, women who breast-fed their infants had a significantly lower rate of relapse than women who did not.

STUDY CONCLUSIONS

In women with MS, the rate of relapse declines during pregnancy, especially in the third trimester, and increases during the first 3 months postpartum before returning to the prepregnancy rate. The overall rate of disability progression does not change over the period studied.

COMMENTARY

At the time of publication, this was the largest prospective analysis on the natural history of pregnancy in MS published. Prior to this study, the influence of pregnancy on the course of MS was controversial, and many women with MS were discouraged from having children out of fear that pregnancy would worsen their disease course. After the publication of this study, the way in which women with MS were counseled about pregnancy changed dramatically.

The significant decrease in clinical attacks in later pregnancy has been confirmed in several prospective clinical trials. Since this trial, the 3-month period of increased risk postpartum has been a consistent observation. The most consistently identified markers associated with postpartum activity are high relapse rate in the year before pregnancy, higher disability level before pregnancy, and relapse during pregnancy.

Question

Does the rate of MS relapse decrease during pregnancy and increase in the postpartum state?

Answer

Yes, the rate of relapse declines during pregnancy, especially in the third trimester, and increases during the first 3 months postpartum before returning to the prepregnancy rate.

Nagagopal Venna ■ Christopher Doughty

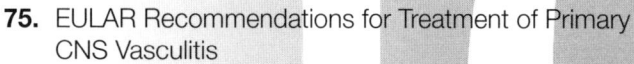

CHAPTER 75	# EULAR RECOMMENDATIONS FOR TREATMENT OF PRIMARY CNS VASCULITIS

EULAR Recommendations for the Management of Primary Small and Medium Vessel Vasculitis

Mukhtyar C, Guillevin L, Cid MC, et al. *Annals Rheum Dis*. 2009;68:310–317

BACKGROUND
Primary angiitis of the CNS (PACNS) refers to vasculitis that is confined to the CNS, without other significant systemic symptoms. PACNS is rare and can be difficult to diagnose, and thus few studies are available to guide treatment. This set of consensus recommendations offered a standardized approach to vasculitis that might be applied to PACNS.

OBJECTIVES
To compile consensus expert recommendations for the evaluation and management of small-and medium-vessel vasculitis.

METHODS
A panel of experts including physicians, immunologists, an epidemiologist, and a drug regulatory expert identified topics for a systematic literature review regarding the evaluation and management of small- and medium-vessel vasculitis and then used the results to generate a series of consensus recommendations.

Patients
NA

Interventions
NA

Outcomes
The literature review and subsequent recommendations focused on the initial work-up, best remission-inducing regimen, choice of therapy for maintenance of remission, management of relapsing or refractory disease, monitoring and follow-up of patients, and complications of therapy. The findings were assimilated into 15 recommendations and assigned a strength of recommendation (SOR) A to D based upon the level of evidence of the studies from which they are derived.

KEY RESULTS
- Serum testing for antineutrophil cytoplasmic antibody (ANCA) using immunofluorescence (SOR A) and tissue biopsy for pathologic assessment (SOR C) are recommended for the evaluation of suspected vasculitis.

- A combination of cyclophosphamide (either IV pulse or daily oral) and high-dose glucocorticoids is recommended for induction of remission (SOR A). A prior meta-analysis of patients with ANCA-associated vasculitis concluded that pulsed cyclophosphamide was more likely to result in remission and less likely to cause adverse effects than daily oral therapy.[1]
- Remission maintenance therapy should consist of a combination of low-dose glucocorticoids and either azathioprine (SOR A), leflunomide (SOR B), or methotrexate (SOR B) for at least 18 months (see Table 75.1).
- Renal function, CBC, liver function tests (LFTs), and inflammatory markers should be checked frequently to assess disease activity, monitor for complications, and guide dose adjustment of immunosuppressants. Periodic urinalysis is essential in patients with exposure to cyclophosphamide, given the risk of hemorrhagic cystitis and bladder cancer.

STUDY CONCLUSIONS

The recommendations provided offer a framework that should apply to the majority of patients with small- and medium-vessel vasculitis, but ongoing research including adequately powered randomized control trials is essential.

COMMENTARY

Prior to this review, a standardized approach to vasculitis affecting the CNS, especially PACNS, was lacking in the literature. An exceptional number of publications were reviewed and offer an excellent foundation for the recommendations generated. Although this study was not specifically designed to address PACNS, the recommendations presented—especially those regarding induction of remission—have been widely adopted into clinical practice. There have been no randomized control trials for the therapy of PACNS, and accordingly these recommendations remain the most comprehensive evidence base available to guide practice. It is worth noting, however, that there remains some variation in practice for the specific treatment of PACNS.

Table 75.1 Options for Remission Maintenance Therapy

Drug	Standard Dosing	Considerations
Prednisone	At least 10 mg/day	Recommended for all patients in addition to one of the following agents.
Azathioprine	2 mg/kg/day	Efficacy equivalent to cyclophosphamide, but safer for remission maintenance.
Methotrexate	20–25 mg/kg/week	Caution and dose adjustment required if renal dysfunction. Ascites/pleural effusions limit elimination.
Leflunomide	20–30 mg/day	May be more effective than methotrexate, but associated with more adverse events.

Question

Is there an adequate evidence base to support a standardized approach to the management of vasculitis affecting the CNS?

Answer

Yes, although there have been no RCTs to assess therapy of PACNS, observations from across the spectrum of small- and medium-vessel vasculitides can be used to generate well-supported expert recommendations that may be applied to vasculitis affecting the CNS.

Reference

1. de Groot K, Adu D, Savage CO. The value of pulse cyclophosphamide in ANCA-associated vasculitis: meta-analysis and critical review. *Nephrol Dial Transplant.* 2001;16:2018–2027.

CHAPTER 76

NMDA-AB RECEPTOR ENCEPHALITIS WITH OVARIAN TERATOMA

Paraneoplastic Anti-*N*-methyl-*D*-aspartate Receptor Encephalitis Associated with Ovarian Teratoma

Dalmau J, Tuzun E, Wu H, et al. *Ann Neurol*. 2007;61(1):25–36

BACKGROUND

Prior to this study, autoimmune encephalitis had been recognized as a paraneoplastic manifestation of multiple cancers. However, cases were generally reported in older patients, and the syndromes were considered to be poorly responsive to treatment with either immunotherapy or removal of the offending tumor. The authors of this study had recently reported five cases of a unique and aggressive autoimmune encephalitis in young women associated with ovarian teratoma that seemed to be responsive to treatment. Through the identification and study of additional patients, the authors were able to identify the target autoantigen of the immune response.

OBJECTIVES

To report the clinical features and autoantigen of a previously unrecognized category of treatment-responsive paraneoplastic encephalitis.

METHODS

Case-control analysis of prototypic cases identified by the authors.

Patients

Twelve women, aged 14 to 44 years, all with autoimmune encephalitis and associated teratomas. The sera and CSF of 200 people, some healthy volunteers and some patients with other causes of encephalitis, served as controls.

Interventions

CSF/serum of patients and controls were assessed with immunohistochemical techniques, utilizing rat tissue with cells expressing the *N*-methyl-*D*-aspartate (NMDA) receptor (NMDAR).

Outcomes

Immunohistochemistry results, as well as common clinical, laboratory, and radiologic findings and treatment response for the patients, were reported.

KEY RESULTS

- A distinct clinical syndrome was described, characterized by a viral-like prodrome and early psychiatric symptoms. Patients later developed seizures and depressed level of consciousness. Several patients developed abnormal movements, autonomic instability, or both.

- CSF analysis demonstrated lymphocytic pleocytosis (9 to 219 cells/µL, median 24 cells/µL) in all patients.
- Neurologic symptoms preceded the diagnosis of teratoma in 11 patients. Eleven teratomas were ovarian, but one was located in the anterior mediastinum.
- Six of seven patients treated with immunosuppression and tumor resection and two patients treated with resection alone improved. Two of three patients treated with immunosuppression alone experienced ongoing neurologic decline and died.
- The sera and CSF of all patients—but no controls—reacted with a subunit of the NMDAR, expressed on the cell surface primarily in the hippocampus. Of the five teratomas available for pathologic review, all expressed this NMDAR subunit. Antibody titers in patients improved with treatment.

STUDY CONCLUSIONS

The study identifies a severe but treatment-responsive form of autoimmune encephalitis in young women with teratoma that is associated with autoantibodies against the NMDAR. The results demonstrate that autoimmunity can affect behavior, emotion, memory, and consciousness.

COMMENTARY

By identifying a common autoantigen for a group of young women with characteristic psychiatric and neurologic syndrome, this study solidified the concept that a clinical syndrome can be highly predictive of a specific autoimmune etiology—and even the specific underlying tumor. Furthermore, this study demonstrated that assessment of NMDAR antibodies could be used as a reliable diagnostic test in patients with the prototypic presentation. Because of the good prognosis associated with early initiation of treatment, expert recommendations now suggest that appropriate first-line immunotherapy—steroids, IV immunoglobulin (IVIG), or plasmapheresis in the case of NMDAR encephalitis—should be initiated, and appropriate screening for malignancy be undertaken even before antibody testing returns when a characteristic clinical syndrome is encountered.[1,2] In the decade since this publication, recognition of NMDAR encephalitis has exploded, and it has been shown to be the most common cause of autoimmune encephalitis worldwide, occurring in additional, diverse clinical settings. Perhaps most importantly, this study emphasized that there are likely many causes of autoimmune encephalitis yet to be discovered.

Question

Can autoimmune encephalitis occur as a paraneoplastic manifestation of previously unrecognized tumors in young patients?

Answer

Yes, a treatable syndrome of acute psychiatric symptoms followed by seizures and depressed consciousness occurs in young female patients with occult teratoma and is associated with autoantibodies against the NMDAR.

References

1. Graus F, Titulaer MJ, Balu R, et al. A clinical approach to diagnosis of autoimmune encephalitis. *Lancet Neurol.* 2016;15:391–1404.
2. Titulaer MJ, McCracken L, Gabilondo I, et al. Treatment and prognostic factors for long-term outcome in patients with anti-*N*-methyl-*D*-aspartate (NMDA) receptor encephalitis: a cohort study. *Lancet Neurol.* 2013;12(2):157–165.

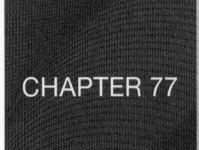

IDENTIFICATION OF SJOGREN'S SYNDROME ASSOCIATED GANGLIONOPATHY

CHAPTER 77

Ataxic Sensory Neuropathy and Dorsal Root Ganglionitis Associated with Sjögren's Syndrome

Griffin JW, Cornblath DR, Alexander E, et al. *Ann Neurol.* 1990;27:304–315

BACKGROUND
A syndrome of sensory neuron degeneration—referred to as sensory ganglionopathy—had previously been described in patients both with and without underlying carcinoma characterized pathologically by lymphocytic infiltration of dorsal root ganglia, suggesting an autoimmune etiology. Several case reports had also suggested an association between sensory ganglionopathy and Sjögren syndrome, predominantly in women, with a suspected autoimmune pathogenesis also involving the dorsal root ganglion. Prior to this study, however, a comprehensive investigation regarding common clinical features and pathologic findings had not been offered.

OBJECTIVES
To demonstrate the relationship between Sjögren syndrome and sensory ganglionopathy by describing the clinical features and pathologic findings in a series of patients presenting with loss of kinesthesia and proprioception as well as sicca symptoms.

METHODS
An observational case series of patients followed at three US academic medical centers between 1984 and 1990.

Patients
Patients presenting with symptoms of predominantly sensory and autonomic neuropathy were screened for findings of sicca syndrome. Patients were included if they had a positive result on the Schirmer's test and positive results on either lip biopsy or serologic testing suggestive of Sjögren syndrome. Thirteen patients, 11 females—aged 36 to 76, met criteria for inclusion.

Interventions
Clinical assessment, electrodiagnostic studies, autonomic function testing, serologic testing, imaging studies to screen for malignancy, and biopsies of sural nerves (in 12 patients) and dorsal root ganglia (in three patients) were performed.

Outcomes
The clinical course of patients, some receiving treatment and some not, was described.

KEY RESULTS

- Sensory abnormalities, dominated by loss of proprioceptive and kinesthetic sensibility, were seen in all patients, with variable anatomic distribution and variable clinical course. Autonomic abnormalities were common but often asymptomatic.
- Only one patient had a preexisting diagnosis of Sjögren syndrome.
- Electrodiagnostic studies demonstrated predominant involvement of sensory nerve fibers in a non-length-dependent pattern, with absent or reduced sensory nerve action potential (SNAP) amplitudes but relatively preserved conduction velocities.
- Nerve biopsies showed a preferential loss of large myelinated fibers, and dorsal root ganglion biopsies showed prominent mononuclear cell infiltrates around individual neurons.
- Ten patients received immunosuppressive medications, but only one patient showed a convincing response to treatment.

STUDY CONCLUSIONS

There is an association between sensory ganglionopathy and features of Sjögren syndrome. An autoimmune pathogenesis is likely, given the inflammatory infiltrate found in dorsal root ganglia.

COMMENTARY

This study attempted to solidify the association between symptoms of sensory ganglionopathy and Sjögren syndrome suggested by several prior case reports. By evaluating patients presenting with suggestive neurologic symptoms, the authors demonstrated that it is important to screen for Sjögren syndrome because sicca symptoms can be quite mild or even absent, and patients usually do not carry a preexisting diagnosis. A striking female predominance was also shown, in accordance with case series published before and after this study. Since the publication of this study, an association has been found between sensory ganglionopathy and other autoimmune diseases such as Rheumatoid Arthritis, Systemic Lupus Erythematosus, and autoimmune hepatitis. Steroids and IVIG have since been reported to be beneficial in select patients, but no randomized control trials have been performed.[1]

Question

Is there an association between sensory ganglionopathy and Sjögren syndrome?

Answer

Yes, patients with symptoms suggestive of a sensory ganglionopathy are often found to have previously unrecognized Sjögren syndrome, with an autoimmune pathogenesis likely underlying the neurologic syndrome.

Reference

1. Takahashi Y, Takata T, Hoshino M, et al. Benefit of IVIG for long-standing ataxic sensory neuronopathy with Sjögren's syndrome. *Neurology.* 2003;60:503–505.

CHAPTER 78

IVIG FOR STIFF PERSON SYNDROME

High-Dose Intravenous Immune Globulin for Stiff Person Syndrome

Dalakas MC, Fujii M, Li M, et al. *NEJM.* 2001;345(26):1870–1876

BACKGROUND

Stiff person syndrome is a rare but disabling disorder characterized by rigidity of truncal and proximal limb muscles and superimposed muscle spasms. At the time of this study, the cause was unknown, but an autoimmune pathogenesis was suspected because of its frequent association with other autoimmune disorders and the characteristic antibodies against glutamic acid decarboxylase (GAD65) found in patients. Gamma-Aminobutyric acid (GABA) agonists such as diazepam and baclofen had been used with symptomatic benefit, but escalating doses were often required, leading to intolerable side effects. Case reports had suggested that treatment with prednisone, IV immune globulin (IVIG), or plasmapheresis might be beneficial.

OBJECTIVES

To determine the efficacy of IVIG for the treatment of stiff person syndrome based on symptomatic measures of stiffness and muscle spasms.

METHODS

Randomized, double-blind, placebo-controlled trial with crossover design conducted at the National Institute of Health from 1996 to 1999.

Patients

Sixteen patients were enrolled. Inclusion criteria: rigidity of limb and axial muscles, clinical and electrophysiological evidence of continuous contraction of agonist/antagonist muscles, episodic spasms, and positive anti-GAD65 antibody testing. Patients were excluded if they were bedridden, had coronary artery disease, IgA deficiency, or renal impairment. All patients were taking benzodiazepines.

Interventions

Half the patients were started on 2 g/kg of IVIG given over 2 days each month for 3 months, and half were started on placebo. After a 1-month washout period, the placebo and treatment arms completed the alternate 3-month arm.

Outcomes

The distribution-of-stiffness index, measuring the anatomic extent of stiffness, and the heightened-sensitivity scale, measuring the number of triggers for muscle spasms, were the primary outcome measures. GAD-65 antibody titers and measures of gait were also monitored.

KEY RESULTS

- IVIG led to significantly lower scores on the distribution-of-stiffness index and the heightened-sensitivity scale. An objective response to treatment was seen in 11 of 16 patients.
- Time required to walk 9.1 m was also significantly decreased, and several of the patients were able to walk unassisted for the first time in years.
- Anti-GAD65 antibody titers declined significantly with IVIG treatment, but did not correlate with disease severity or response to treatment.
- All patients were able to tolerate the planned 3-month therapy.

STUDY CONCLUSIONS

IVIG is a safe and effective treatment for stiff person syndrome, leading to a reduction in stiffness and propensity for muscle spasms and allowing for an increased ability to perform the activities of daily living.

COMMENTARY

This study was the first randomized control trial to demonstrate efficacy of an immunologic therapy for stiff person syndrome. The small size and the lack of formal reporting of safety data are relative limitations of this study, but this remains the only randomized control trial for immunotherapy in stiff person syndrome. It is now widely accepted that stiff person syndrome is an autoimmune condition, with accumulating evidence that anti-GAD65 antibodies impair the synthesis of GABA, though not all patients with stiff person syndrome have detectable anti-GAD65 antibodies. Observational data from nonrandomized trials have since suggested that plasmapheresis, corticosteroids, rituximab, and other oral immunosuppressive agents may also be beneficial in patients with stiff person syndrome. Nevertheless, the clinical course of stiff person syndrome remains highly variable, and some patients with the disorder will continue with ongoing disability despite trials of many of the established treatments.

Question

Is IVIG an effective treatment for stiff person syndrome?

Answer

Yes, monthly infusion of IVIG reduces both stiffness and muscle spasms in patients with stiff person syndrome and may lead to improved ability to independently perform the activities of daily living in some patients.

EPILEPSY

M. Brandon Westover ■ Anna M. Bank

CHAPTER 79

LORAZEPAM FOR TREATMENT OF STATUS EPILEPTICUS

A Comparison of Four Treatments for Generalized Convulsive Status Epilepticus

Treiman DM, Meyers PD, Walton NY, et al. *NEJM*. 1998;339(12):792–798

BACKGROUND

Status epilepticus is a life-threatening neurologic emergency, and treatment should be initiated early and aggressively. While many drugs are effective in terminating seizures, the best first-line antiepileptic drug (AED) for the treatment of status epilepticus was unknown prior to this study.

OBJECTIVES

To determine which IV AED is most effective in terminating status epilepticus.

METHODS

Randomized trial conducted at 16 Veterans Affairs medical centers and 6 affiliated university hospitals in the United States from 1990 to 1995.

Patients

518 patients with overt or subtle status epilepticus were included in the final study analysis. Overt status epilepticus (384 patients) was defined as two or more generalized convulsions without recovery of consciousness in-between or 10 minutes of ongoing convulsions. Subtle status epilepticus (134 patients) was defined as coma with ictal discharges on electroencephalopgraphy (EEG), with or without subtle convulsive movements. Patients were included if they met criteria for status epilepticus at the time of enrollment, regardless of prior AED treatment.

Interventions

Patients were randomized to treatment with diazepam followed by phenytoin (131 patients), phenytoin alone (127 patients), lorazepam (136 patients), or phenobarbital (124 patients). Patients and physicians were blind to AED selection.

Outcomes

The primary outcome was successful treatment of status epilepticus (defined as cessation of all clinical and electrographic seizure activity within 20 minutes after the start of infusion), without recurrence of clinical or electrographic seizure activity within 60 minutes. Secondary outcomes included seizure recurrence within 12 hours, recovery of consciousness within 12 hours, hospital discharge within 30 days, and 30-day mortality rate.

KEY RESULTS

- Across all patients, lorazepam was effective more often than phenytoin. This difference was entirely accounted for by patients with overt status epilepticus.
- Across treatment groups, initial treatment was more likely to be effective in patients with overt status epilepticus than in patients with subtle status epilepticus (55.5% vs. 14.9%).
- Status epilepticus was less likely to recur within 12 hours in patients with overt status epilepticus than in patients with subtle status epilepticus (11.3% vs. 20.0%).
- Patients with overt status epilepticus were more likely to regain consciousness within 12 hours than patients with subtle status epilepticus (17.4% vs. 0.0%)
- Although there were no significant differences in 30-day discharge outcomes across treatments, patients responding to the initial treatment were more likely to be discharged within 30 days. Mortality was twice as high in the subtle status epilepticus group (64.7% vs. 27.0%).

STUDY CONCLUSIONS

Lorazepam is more effective than phenytoin when used as the initial treatment for patients with overt status epilepticus. Patients with overt status epilepticus achieve more frequent and longer-lasting seizure control and have a lower mortality rate than patients with subtle status epilepticus.

COMMENTARY

This was the first randomized, double-blind trial to compare initial treatments for status epilepticus. In part because of this study, which demonstrated that lorazepam was more effective than phenytoin, experts now recommend benzodiazepines as initial therapy for status epilepticus. Of note, three of the most commonly used IV AEDs—valproate, levetiracetam, and lacosamide—were not included in this study. The 2012 Neurocritical Care Society "Guidelines for the Evaluation and Management of Status Epilepticus" recommend benzodiazepines (IV lorazepam or intramuscular [IM] midazolam) for first-line emergent treatment of status epilepticus because of their efficacy, rapid onset, and ease of administration. This study was also one of the first to demonstrate that patients with subtle (now referred to as nonconvulsive) status epilepticus have a worse prognosis than patients with convulsive status epilepticus.

Question

Is there a single best initial treatment for status epilepticus?

Answer

No, many agents are comparably effective in the treatment of status epilepticus, but benzodiazepines such as lorazepam should be administered first.

CHAPTER 80

MAGNESIUM FOR THE PREVENTION OF ECLAMPSIA

A Comparison of Magnesium Sulfate with Phenytoin for the Prevention of Eclampsia

Lucas MJ, Leveno KJ, Cunningham FG. *NEJM*. 1995;333(4):201–205

BACKGROUND

Preeclampsia is a hypertensive disorder of pregnancy that poses life-threatening risks to both the mother and the fetus. Eclampsia is the presence of generalized tonic-clonic seizures in a patient with preeclampsia. Eclamptic seizures have historically been managed with magnesium sulfate based on observational data, but prior to this study, no randomized trial had compared the efficacy of magnesium sulfate and AEDs for the prevention of seizures in patients with preeclampsia.

OBJECTIVES

To compare the efficacy of magnesium sulfate and phenytoin for the prevention of eclampsia in patients with preeclampsia.

METHODS

Randomized trial at one academic medical center in the United States from 1993 to 1994.

Patients

2,138 patients who were admitted to the labor and delivery unit, with systolic blood pressure above 140 and diastolic blood pressure above 90, gave consent for study participation. Patients were excluded if they were about to give birth, had already given birth, or if they had a prior diagnosis of epilepsy or presented with eclamptic seizures. 1,049 patients were randomized to the magnesium group and 1,089 were randomized to the phenytoin group.

Interventions

Patients were randomized to treatment with IM magnesium sulfate or IV phenytoin. All patients who developed eclampsia were treated with magnesium. Neither patients nor physicians were blind to group assignment.

Outcomes

The primary outcome was a diagnosis of eclampsia, defined as a witnessed generalized tonic-clonic seizure.

KEY RESULTS

- Eclampsia occurred significantly more frequently in patients treated with phenytoin than in patients treated with magnesium (10 patients vs. 0 patients).

STUDY CONCLUSIONS

Magnesium is superior to phenytoin for the prevention of eclampsia in patients with preeclampsia.

COMMENTARY

The purpose of this study was to determine the optimal agent for preventing eclampsia in patients with preeclampsia. Although magnesium had historically been used for this purpose, this was the first study to demonstrate that it is superior to a traditional AED and confirmed its standing as the gold standard. One caveat is that phenytoin was the only traditional AED compared to magnesium in this study, and it is possible that other AEDs may produce results comparable to magnesium. The 2014 American College of Obstetricians and Gynecologists "Hypertension in Pregnancy" Task Force Recommendation suggests treating patients with severe preeclampsia (blood pressure >160/110, thrombocytopenia, or evidence of end-organ dysfunction) with magnesium to prevent eclampsia.

Question

Should magnesium sulfate be given to patients with preeclampsia to prevent eclampsia?

Answer

Yes, magnesium sulfate should be the treatment of choice for patients with preeclampsia.

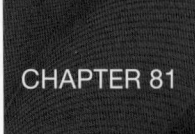

ANTIEPILEPTIC DRUG TREATMENT AFTER A FIRST UNPROVOKED SEIZURE

CHAPTER 81

Randomized Clinical Trial on the Efficacy of Antiepileptic Drugs in Reducing the Risk of Relapse after a First Unprovoked Tonic-Clonic Seizure

First Seizure Trial Group. *Neurology*. 1993; 43(3): 478–483

BACKGROUND

Many patients will have one unprovoked seizure, but only half of them will develop epilepsy. Because AEDs often have adverse side effects, and many patients will not have further seizures, AED treatment is often not initiated after a first seizure. Prior to this study, the difference in seizure recurrence rates between patients who initiate AED treatment immediately after a first seizure and those who do not was unknown.

OBJECTIVES

To compare the risk of seizure recurrence between patients who initiate AED treatment immediately after a first seizure and those who do not.

METHODS

Randomized trial conducted at 35 university and hospital centers in Italy from 1988 to 1991.

Patients

397 patients ranging from 2 to 70 years of age were randomized within 7 days of a first unprovoked generalized tonic-clonic seizure. Patients with a first unprovoked partial seizure, multiple seizures within 24 hours, status epilepticus, a seizure within 30 days of an acute neurologic injury (i.e., stroke, head trauma, CNS infection), toxic or metabolic disturbance, or known neurologic or psychiatric illness were excluded. 204 patients were randomized to immediate treatment and 193 were not.

Interventions

Patients were randomized to immediate AED treatment or to treatment only after a recurrent seizure. AEDs included carbamazepine, phenytoin, phenobarbital, and valproate. AED selection was made by the treating physician. Neither patients nor physicians were blind to group assignment.

Outcomes

The primary outcome was the occurrence of one or more generalized tonic-clonic seizures, with or without partial onset, during the 2-year follow-up period.

KEY RESULTS

- Seizures were more common in untreated patients than in treated patients (38.9% vs. 17.6%).
- Untreated patients were 2.8 times more likely to have a seizure (hazard ratio 2.8, adjusted for age and presence of epileptiform abnormalities on EEG, 95% CI, 1.9 to 4.2).
- The probability of seizure recurrence among treated patients was 4% by 1 month, 7% by 3 months, 9% by 6 months, 17% by 12 months, 23% by 18 months, and 25% by 24 months.
- The probability of seizure recurrence among untreated patients was 8% by 1 month, 18% by 3 months, 28% by 6 months, 41% by 12 months, 45% by 18 months, and 51% by 24 months.

STUDY CONCLUSIONS

Immediate initiation of AED treatment reduces the risk of seizure recurrence after a first unprovoked generalized tonic seizure.

COMMENTARY

Patients presenting with a first unprovoked seizure are often not started on AED treatment. This was the first randomized trial to directly compare seizure recurrence rates for patients who start immediate AED treatment after a first seizure and those who do not. This study prompted physicians and patients to carefully weigh the higher risk of a second seizure against the risk of adverse drug events. Because the study was not blinded, seizures may have been underreported in the treated group and overreported in the untreated group. The 2015 American Academy of Neurology/American Epilepsy Society guideline "Management of an Unprovoked First Seizure in Adults" encourages physicians to counsel patients that AED treatment is likely to reduce the risk of seizure recurrence in the first 2 years after a first seizure. The decision to start an AED after first unprovoked seizure is made with various considerations in place by both the physician and the patient together, accounting for the patient's occupational hazards, living circumstances, and degree of interference with daily life.

Question

Should AED treatment be initiated after a first unprovoked generalized tonic-clonic seizure?

Answer

Yes, if the physician and the patient determine that the adverse effects of a second seizure outweigh the adverse effects of AED treatment.

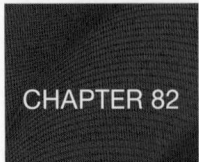

CHAPTER 82

INTRAVENOUS VS. INTRAMUSCULAR BENZODIAZEPINES FOR STATUS EPILEPTICUS

Intramuscular versus Intravenous Therapy for Prehospital Status Epilepticus
Silbergleit R, Durkalski V, Lowenstein D, et al. *NEJM*. 2012;366(7):591–600

BACKGROUND
Benzodiazepines are the best first-line treatment for status epilepticus, and early cessation of seizures has been shown to improve patient outcomes. Because IV access can be difficult to obtain prior to emergency department arrival and during convulsions, many patients are treated intramuscularly. This study was the first to compare the efficacy of IV and IM benzodiazepines in treating status epilepticus.

OBJECTIVES
Noninferiority trial to determine whether IM midazolam is as effective as IV lorazepam in treating status epilepticus.

METHODS
Randomized trial conducted in 33 emergency medical service agencies and 79 receiving hospitals in the United States from 2009 to 2011.

Patients
893 patients whose convulsions lasted for at least 5 minutes and persisted after paramedic arrival, or who had intermittent convulsions over a 5-minute period without regaining consciousness. Patients were excluded if the acute precipitant of the seizures was trauma, hypoglycemia, cardiac arrest, or bradycardia. 445 patients were randomized to treatment with lorazepam, and 448 were randomized to treatment with IM midazolam.

Interventions
Patients were randomized to treatment with IM midazolam followed by IV placebo, or IM placebo followed by IV lorazepam. If IV access could not be obtained within 10 minutes, the IV intervention was delivered intraosseously, and this was considered to be equivalent to IV delivery. Patients and paramedics were blind to group assignment.

Outcomes
The primary outcome was cessation of seizures prior to emergency department arrival without administration of rescue therapy. Secondary outcomes included time from randomization to termination of convulsions, time from active drug administration to termination of convulsions, floor or ICU admission, duration of hospitalization, intubation, and recurrence of seizures within 12 hours.

KEY RESULTS

- Midazolam was effective in terminating seizures significantly more often than lorazepam (73.4% vs. 63.4% of patients).
- Fewer patients in the midazolam group were admitted to the hospital.
- All other secondary outcomes were similar between groups.

STUDY CONCLUSIONS

IM midazolam is more effective than IV lorazepam in terminating status epilepticus.

COMMENTARY

IM midazolam is easier to administer than IV lorazepam, but prior to the RAM-PART (Rapid Anticonvulsant Medication Prior to Arrival Trial), it was unknown whether it was as effective in treating status epilepticus. Not only was midazolam noninferior to lorazepam, it also met statistical standards for superiority. Although use of midazolam had already begun to increase in practice, its use was validated by this trial. The 2012 Neurocritical Care Society "Guidelines for the Evaluation and Management of Status Epilepticus" currently recommend benzodiazepines (IV lorazepam or IM midazolam) as first-line emergent treatment of status epilepticus.

Question

Can IM midazolam be used for the treatment of status epilepticus?

Answer

Yes, it is just as effective if not more effective as IV lorazepam and it is easier to administer.

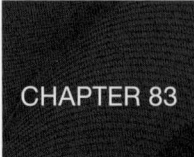

CONTINUOUS EEG MONITORING FOR EVALUATION OF NONCONVULSIVE STATUS EPILEPTICUS

CHAPTER 83

Detection of Electrographic Seizures with Continuous EEG Monitoring in Critically Ill Patients

Claassen J, Mayer SA, Kowalski RG, et al. *Neurology*. 2004;62:1743–1748

BACKGROUND

Seizures and status epilepticus are common in patients with acute neurologic conditions, but they are not always clinically evident. Recognizing and treating these seizures reduces metabolic demand on already damaged brain tissue. Prior to this study, it was not known how long to continue EEG monitoring in patients where there was a clinical suspicion for seizures to begin with.

OBJECTIVES

To identify patients at high risk for electrographic seizures following acute neurologic injury, and to identify patients who may require longer EEG monitoring in order to capture seizure activity.

METHODS

This was a retrospective observational study at a single academic medical center in the United States between 1996 and 2002.

Patients

570 patients underwent continuous EEG monitoring for unexplained decreased level of consciousness or suspected subclinical seizures. Patients were excluded if they underwent continuous EEG monitoring for IV AED titration for status epilepticus, or IV phenobarbital titration for increased intracranial pressure.

Interventions

Patients were preselected based on presence or absence of continuous EEG monitoring. No prespecified duration of EEG monitoring, or clinical inclusion criterion other than decreased level of consciousness or suspected subclinical seizures, was utilized.

Outcomes

The primary outcome was the presence of electrographic seizures on continuous EEG monitoring. Secondary outcomes were the time to first seizure, the presence of a first seizure after 24 hours of continuous EEG monitoring, the seizure pattern, and death or disability status at the time of hospital discharge.

KEY RESULTS

- Nineteen percent of patients had electrographic seizures, 92% of whom had exclusively nonconvulsive seizures.
- Eighty-eight percent of patients with seizures had their first seizure during the first 24 hours of monitoring, whereas 5% had their first seizure between 24 and 48 hours after the start of monitoring, and 7% had their first seizure more than 48 hours after the start of monitoring.
- Coma, age <18 years, history of epilepsy, and convulsive seizures prior to initiation of continuous EEG monitoring were independent predictors of electrographic seizures.
- Periodic lateralized epileptiform discharges, generalized periodic epileptiform discharges, and burst-suppression were more likely to be recorded in patients with seizures than in those without; however, there was no reported temporal relationship to seizures themselves.

STUDY CONCLUSIONS

Seizures occur often in patients with acute neurologic injury and are usually nonconvulsive. Patients may require more than 24 hours of continuous EEG monitoring before the first seizure is recorded.

COMMENTARY

Nonconvulsive seizures are common in patients with acute neurologic injury, and these may occur more than 24 hours after the beginning of continuous EEG monitoring. Many institutions now monitor patients for 24 or 48 hours. It is important to note that this was a retrospective study, and patients were selected to undergo EEG monitoring because of a decline in mental status or suspicion for subclinical seizures. The duration of continuous EEG monitoring varied extensively among the patient population, and the analysis does not account for early cessation of EEG monitoring in patients prior to a captured seizure. The absence of any prespecified duration of monitoring remains a major limitation of the study. The 2012 Neurocritical Care Society "Guidelines for the Evaluation and Management of Status Epilepticus" currently recommend continuous EEG monitoring for all patients with recent convulsive status, coma, intracranial hemorrhage, epileptiform abnormalities on routine EEG, or suspected nonconvulsive seizures. There is ongoing uncertainty regarding which patient's would most benefit from continuous EEG monitoring and which EEG patterns warrant aggressive vs. conservative management.

Question

Should all patients with acute neurologic injury and a decline in mental status undergo continuous EEG monitoring?

Answer

Yes, because seizures frequently occur in this population and are almost always nonconvulsive.

SECTION 12

HEADACHE AND PAIN

William Mullally ■ Sheena Chew

CHAPTER 84

SUMATRIPTAN FOR MIGRAINE

Treatment of Migraine Attacks with Sumatriptan

The Subcutaneous Sumatriptan International Study Group. *NEJM*. 1991;325:316–321

BACKGROUND

This study evaluated subcutaneous sumatriptan for treatment of migraine headache. Prior to this study, there were no RCTs for the treatment of acute migraine headache, and recommendations for migraine treatment were based on clinical experience alone. Ergotamine was the most widely accepted pharmacologic treatment for acute migraine treatment, but its use was limited by its side effect profile. Subcutaneous sumatriptan was evaluated instead of IV sumatriptan because IV sumatriptan produced the unacceptable adverse side effect of coronary vasoconstriction.

OBJECTIVES

To determine whether subcutaneous sumatriptan is a well-tolerated and effective treatment for acute migraine headache.

METHODS

Randomized, double-blinded, placebo-controlled, parallel-group clinical trial, carried out in 1989 with 639 patients enrolled from 58 hospitals in 10 countries.

Patients

Patients were men and women aged 18 to 65 (96% white) who met International Headache Society criteria for migraine with or without aura. Notable exclusion critera included history of heart disease, peripheral vascular disease, stroke, seizures, hypertension, pregnancy, use of opiates or ergot-containing medications, or use of analgesics within 6 hours of study enrollment.

Interventions

At the time of a migraine attack, patients who rated their headaches as moderate or severe were randomly assigned an injection of placebo, 6 mg sumatriptan, or 8 mg sumatriptan. After 60 minutes, a second injection of either placebo or 6 mg sumatriptan was given if the patient was not completely free of pain.

Outcomes

The primary endpoints were (1) the proportion of patients with improvement in the severity of headache and (2) the proportion of patients with complete resolution of pain. Headache pain was measured on a scale of 0 to 3 completed by the subject: 0 = no pain, 1 = mild pain, 2 = moderate pain, and 3 = severe pain. Headache pain was considered "improved" after treatment if the patient's headache rating decreased from 2–3 to 0–1 and considered "resolved" if rating decreased to 0.

KEY RESULTS

- The proportion of patients who reported improvement in headache severity was approximately 50% higher in the sumatriptan group compared to the placebo group ($p < 0.001$).
- Complete resolution of pain occurred in a significantly higher proportion of patients treated with either 6 or 8 mg sumatriptan compared to placebo ($p < 0.001$).
- Treatment with sumatriptan also led to significant relief of migraine-associated symptoms, resolution of functional disability, reduced need for rescue medication at 120 minutes, and reduced migraine recurrence.
- There was no significant difference in effect between sumatriptan treatment regimens (6 mg once, 8 mg once, or 6 mg twice).
- Most adverse events were mild and self-resolved within 10 to 30 minutes. Common adverse events included injection-site reaction, nausea or vomiting flushing, abnormal sensation, dizziness, paresthesias, and headache.

STUDY CONCLUSIONS

A single 6 mg dose of subcutaneous sumatriptan is a safe and effective treatment for acute migraine.

COMMENTARY

Prior to this study, acute migraine treatment was based on clinical experience because there were no RCTs of pharmacologic therapies for migraine in the literature. The sumatriptan study was the first placebo-controlled clinical trial to demonstrate an effective and well-tolerated pharmacologic treatment for acute migraine headache. It opened the door to the use of other triptan medications for migraine treatment. The major limitation of this study is its generalizability because study subjects were 96% white and without any major medical comorbidities. It also excluded individuals who had taken other medications for headache, so it did not define its efficacy against other analgesics. The study was also sponsored by Glaxo Research Group, maker of Imitrex.

Question

Is sumatriptan an effective treatment for acute migraine headache?

Answer

Yes. A single dose of 6 mg sumatriptan administered via subcutaneous injection is an effective and generally well-tolerated treatment for acute migraine in individuals without other medical morbidities.

CHAPTER 85

TOPIRAMATE FOR MIGRAINE PREVENTION

Topiramate for Migraine Prevention: A Randomized Controlled Trial

Brandes J, Saper JR, Diamond M, et al. *JAMA*. 2004;291(8):965–973

BACKGROUND

This seminal study added topiramate to the list of first-line migraine prophylactic agents. Prior small studies suggested that topiramate could be efficacious for migraine prevention, which set the stage for this large multicenter randomized trial.

OBJECTIVES

To determine whether topiramate is well tolerated and effective at preventing migraine headaches.

METHODS

Randomized, double-blind, placebo-controlled, parallel-group clinical trial, conducted in 468 patients from 52 different clinical centers in North America.

Patients

Patients were individuals aged 12 to 65 (87% women, 88% white) who met International Headache Society criteria for migraine with or without aura, had 3 to 12 migraines per 28 days, but no more than 15 headache days per 28 days. Notable exclusion criteria included women of child-bearing age who were not on birth control, headaches other than migraine, tension, or sinus headaches, onset of migraine after 50 years of age, overuse of analgesics, use of other known migraine prophylactic medications (including herbal and vitamin supplementation), and history of renal stones.

Interventions

Patients started the study with a washout period of 2 weeks during which all migraine preventive medications were tapered. Washout was followed by a baseline phase of 4 weeks during which headache frequency and severity were recorded. Patients were then randomized to one of four treatment groups: (1) placebo, (2) topiramate 50 mg/day, (3) topiramate 100 mg/day, or (4) topiramate 200 mg/day. Patients started topiramate at 25 mg/day, and dose was increased by 25 mg/week until patients reached their maximum tolerated dose or assigned dose. Treatment was continued for 18 weeks. Headache frequency, severity, and use of rescue medications were recorded.

Outcomes

The primary endpoint was reduction in average 28-day migraine frequency. Secondary endpoints included: (1) proportion of patients with >50% reduction in migraine frequency; (2) mean change in monthly migraine days, severity, and duration; and (3) change in number of days per month requiring rescue medication.

KEY RESULTS

- There was a significant decrease in the mean monthly migraine frequency in the groups treated with 100 mg/day topiramate (5.8 per month to 3.5 per month) or 200 mg/day topiramate (5.1 per month to 3.0 per month) compared to placebo (5.6 per month to 4.5 per month).
- The topiramate groups had significantly fewer days per month of rescue medication use compared to the placebo group.
- Migraine frequency was significantly reduced for the topiramate groups by month 1 of treatment.
- Patients treated with topiramate had statistically significant decrease in body weight during the trial, when compared to placebo-treated patients.

STUDY CONCLUSIONS

Topiramate, at a target dose of 100 mg/day in two divided doses, is an effective treatment for the prevention of migraine headaches.

COMMENTARY

Prior to this study, the major agents used for migraine prophylaxis were propanolol, amitriptyline, and valproic acid. This study added topiramate to the armamentarium, and topiramate with a target dose of 100 mg/day is now considered one of the first-line medications for migraine prophylaxis. Though this study showed that topiramate 200 mg/day reduced migraine duration more than 100 mg/day, a 2013 Cochrane meta-analysis showed no difference.[1] Weight loss was an unintended side effect of topiramate use. This study is limited by its generalizability, the study population consisted of mostly white women, and combination therapy was not allowed. Johnson & Johnson, manufacturer of Topamax, sponsored the study, paid for independent statistical review, and assisted in the preparation of the manuscript.

Question

Is topiramate a safe and effective medication for prevention of migraine headaches?

Answer

Yes. Topiramate can be started and uptitrated slowly to a target dose of 100 mg/day. Caution should be used in individuals with a history of renal stones and women who may become pregnant.

Reference

1. Linde M, Mulleners WM, Chronicle EP, et al. Topiramate for the prophylaxis of episodic migraine in adults. *Cochrane Database Syst Rev.* 2013(6):CD010610.

DULOXETINE FOR CHEMO-INDUCED PAINFUL NEUROPATHY

CHAPTER 86

Effect of Duloxetine on Pain, Function, and Quality of Life among Patients with Chemotherapy-Induced Painful Peripheral Neuropathy: A Randomized Clinical Trial

Smith E, Pang H, Cirrincione C, et al. *JAMA*. 2013;309(13):1359–1367

BACKGROUND

Chemotherapy-induced painful peripheral neuropathy affects approximately 20% to 40% of patients treated with neurotoxic chemotherapy. Despite its prevalence, there was no known effective pharmacologic therapy until this study.

OBJECTIVES

To determine whether duloxetine is a well-tolerated and effective treatment for painful chemotherapy-induced neuropathy.

METHODS

Double-blind, placebo-controlled, crossover clinical trial, conducted in 231 patients enrolled between 2008 and 2011 through eight separate multicenter research networks throughout the United States.

Patients

Patients were individuals 25 years and older (63% women, 81% white) who (1) had been treated with paclitaxel, oxaliplatin, docetaxel, or cisplatin; (2) had a clinical diagnosis of chemotherapy-induced neuropathy based on symptom history, loss of deep tendon reflexes, or presence of stocking-glove numbness or paresthesias beginning after neurotoxic chemotherapy; (3) had at least grade 1 sensory pain based on National Cancer Institute's Common Terminology Criteria for Adverse Events version 3.0; and (4) reported at least 4 on 10-point scale for average neuropathic pain for at least 3 months after chemotherapy. Exclusion criteria included history of compressive neuropathy, leptomeningeal carcinomatosis, suicidal ideation, bipolar disease, treatment with other neurotoxic chemotherapeutic agents, or use of other drugs known to influence serotonin levels.

Interventions

Patients were randomized to two treatment groups, which were stratified by drug class (taxane vs. platinum) and concomitant use of other analgesics. During the initial treatment phase, Group A received 30 mg duloxetine once daily for 1 week, followed by 60 mg once daily for 4 weeks. Group B received placebo for the entire duration. The initial treatment phase was followed by a washout period of 2 weeks during which neither group received any medications. Patients then underwent a 4-week crossover period, during which Group A received placebo and Group B received duloxetine.

Outcomes
The primary endpoint was average pain over 24 hours, assessed weekly on a scale from 0 to 10. The secondary endpoints included: (1) the degree to which pain interfered with daily activities, (2) patient-reported quality of life, and (3) adverse events.

KEY RESULTS
- During the initial treatment period, there was a significant decrease in the average pain scores in duloxetine-first group compared to placebo-first group. This effect was replicated in the crossover period, when the duloxetine-second group reported decreased average pain compared to the placebo-second group. The decrease in pain score was >10%, which was considered to be clinically meaningful.
- Patients treated with duloxetine had a statistically significant decrease in pain interference with daily function and increase in quality-of-life measurements compared to the placebo group.
- Although the study was not powered to distinguish the effect of duloxetine on neuropathy caused by platinum-based agents vs. taxanes, there was a nonstatistically significant trend toward greater benefit for individuals treated with platinum-based chemotherapy.
- There were no severe adverse events. The most common adverse events included fatigue, insomnia, and nausea.

STUDY CONCLUSIONS
In comparison to placebo, duloxetine treatment provided a statistically and clinically significant decrease in reported pain from chemotherapy-induced neuropathy.

COMMENTARY
This was the first study to demonstrate efficacy of any pharmacologic agent for chemotherapy-induced neuropathy. Of note, the mean change in pain score in patients treated with duloxetine was 1.06 on an 11-point scale. It is difficult to judge whether this degree of improvement will be clinically meaningful to any individual patient, and the benefits of treatment need to be weighed against side effects and long-term drug interactions. For duloxetine, this includes the risk of serotonin syndrome, interaction with CYP P450, interference with warfarin and nonsteroidal antiinflammatory drug (NSAID) metabolism, and inhibition of conversion of tamoxifen to its active metabolite for treatment of breast cancer.

Question
Is duloxetine a safe and effective medication for treatment of chemotherapy-induced painful peripheral neuropathy?

Answer
Yes, at a target dose of 60 mg/day.

CHAPTER 87

PREGABALIN FOR NEUROPATHIC PAIN

Efficacy of Pregabalin in Neuropathic Pain Evaluated in a 12-Week, Randomized, Double-Blind, Multicenter, Placebo-Controlled Trial of Flexible- and Fixed-Dose Regimens

Freynhagen R, Strojek K, Griesing T, et al. *Pain*. 2005;115(3):254–263

BACKGROUND

Painful diabetic peripheral neuropathy and postherpetic neuralgia are common conditions—diabetic neuropathy occurs in approximately 15% of patients with diabetes, and postherpetic neuralgia occurs in approximately 11% of herpes zoster patients. At the time of the study, several agents were used for the treatment of neuropathic pain, including gabapentin, tricyclic antidepressants, and opiates. Despite these options, patients often had refractory symptoms. Prior studies in animal models, as well as small cohort human studies, suggested that pregabalin was effective in reducing neuropathic pain.

OBJECTIVES

To determine whether pregabalin is a well-tolerated and effective treatment for neuropathic pain caused by diabetic neuropathy or postherpetic neuralgia.

METHODS

Randomized, double-blind, placebo-controlled, parallel-group clinical trial, conducted in 338 patients enrolled across 60 clinical centers in 9 European countries.

Patients

Patients were individuals aged 18 or older (54% male, 97.6% white) with a diagnosis of either painful diabetic neuropathy or postherpetic neuralgia and a self-reported pain score of 40 mm or more on visual analogue scale of 0 to 100 mm. Exclusion criteria included pregnancy or lactation, any clinically significant or unstable medical or psychiatric condition, recent malignancy, abnormal EEG, history of severe pain unrelated to neuropathy, evidence of other etiologies of neuropathy including abnormal renal function, hematologic studies, hepatitis B or C, HIV, and any other neurologic diagnosis.

Interventions

Patients first underwent 1 week of observation to establish baseline pain scores. They were subsequently randomized to placebo, flexible-dose pregabalin (150 to 600 mg/day), or fixed-dose pregabalin (600 mg/day). After randomization, they underwent 12 weeks of treatment. The flexible-dose group received escalating doses of pregabalin titrated weekly, based on response and tolerability. The fixed group received 300 mg/day for 1 week, followed by 600 mg/day.

Outcomes

The primary endpoint was the reduction in mean pain score on a scale of 0 to 10. Secondary endpoints included (1) change in sleep interference score, (2) MOS Sleep Scale, and (3) Patient Global Impression of Change scale.

KEY RESULTS

- Compared to placebo, both the fixed- and flexible-dose pregabalin groups experienced significant decreases in pain scores by week 1 or 2 of treatment.
- Number needed to treat for >50% reduction of ongoing pain was 3.8 for all pregabalin-treated patients.
- Both pregabalin groups were superior compared to placebo in improving sleep disturbance.
- Treatment with pregabalin was associated with weight gain and peripheral edema.

STUDY CONCLUSIONS

Twice-daily dosing of pregabalin of a total 300 mg/day is superior to placebo in the treatment of painful diabetic neuropathy and postherpetic neuralgia.

COMMENTARY

Compared to prior pregabalin trials, this study showed that (1) twice-daily dosing of pregabalin is as effective as thrice-daily dosing and (2) flexible uptitration of medication dosing is also efficacious. The major limitation of this study is its generalizability. Individuals who have painful diabetic neuropathy or postherpetic neuralgia in general practice will likely have clinically significant comorbid medical conditions, be taking analgesic medications, and be of a more diverse ethnic background. This study was funded by Pfizer, manufacturer of Lyrica.

Question

Is pregabalin a safe and effective medication for treatment of peripheral neuropathy?

Answer

Yes. Pregabalin, at a target dose of 300 mg/day divided in two daily doses, is effective in treating pain from diabetic neuropathy and postherpetic neuralgia. It is effective within 1 week of reaching the target dose.

CHAPTER 88

AMITRIPTYLINE PROPHYLAXIS FOR HEADACHE

Amitriptyline in the Prophylactic Treatment of Migraine and Chronic Daily Headache

Couch JR; for the Amitriptyline versus Placebo Study Group. *Headache*. 2011;51(1):33–51

BACKGROUND

Amitriptyline was first described as a possible treatment for chronic tension headache in the 1960s. Despite widespread prophylactic use by the early 2000s, there had been no large trials of amitriptyline for migraine prevention.

OBJECTIVES

To evaluate whether amitriptyline is a well-tolerated and effective prophylactic treatment for migraine headache or chronic daily headache.

METHODS

Double-blind, placebo-controlled, parallel-group clinical trial conducted between 1976 and 1979 in 391 patients through 10 different clinical centers in the United States.

Patients

Patients were individuals aged 18 to 70 years (81% female; racial background not noted) who had two or more headaches per month and were diagnosed with primary migraine headaches based on meeting three of five symptomatic criteria. Exclusion criteria included history of headaches secondary to other causes, pregnancy or lactation, use of other antimigraine agents, use of monoamine oxidase inhibitors (MAOIs), history of urinary retention, glaucoma, cardiac disease, hypertension, thyroid disease, and seizure disorder.

Interventions

Patients underwent a 20-week study with three phases: baseline placebo (weeks 1 to 4), randomization and dose titration (week 5 to 8), and maintenance (weeks 9 to 20).

Outcomes

The primary endpoints included (1) headache frequency, measured as number of days per 28 days with a headache of any degree, (2) headache severity, measured on 5-point scale, and (3) headache duration. Secondary endpoints included clinician-reported measure of "impact on patient's life" and self-reported "change since last visit."

KEY RESULTS

- There was no significant reduction in headache severity or duration during the treatment period (weeks 5 to 20) compared to the baseline placebo period (weeks 1 to 4) in either the treatment or the placebo group.

- There was a significant decrease in headache frequency during the treatment period compared to the baseline placebo period for *both* the amitriptyline and placebo groups.
- The amitriptyline arm had increased reports of dry mucous membranes, constipation, urinary retention, dizziness, and somnolence.
- Patients were also subdivided for reanalysis into two groups: chronic daily headache (>16 migraines/month) and intermittent migraine (≤16 migraines/month).
  - For the chronic daily headache group, there was a significant decrease in headache frequency in the amitriptyline-treated arm compared to placebo at both 8 weeks and the end of the study. There was no difference in the intermittent migraine group.

STUDY CONCLUSIONS

Amitriptyline of up to 100 mg/day is superior to placebo for treating chronic daily headache, but not intermittent migraine.

COMMENTARY

This study enrolled patients in the 1970s but was not published until 2010 due to the loss of amitriptyline's patent protection by the study's sponsor (Merck, Sharp, and Dohme Research Laboratories), initial statistical analyses that were not promising, and change in academic position of the lead author. At the time of this study's publication (reevaluation funded by Merck & Co), amitriptyline was one of the most commonly used agents for migraine prophylaxis, and it was considered first-line treatment based on expert opinion and small studies that showed superiority of amitriptyline to placebo or noninferiority compared to other approved migraine prophylactic agents. Overall, findings in this study were mixed. Although there was no difference in the severity or duration of headaches between amitriptyline- and placebo-treated groups, there was an effect on headache frequency in the subgroup with chronic daily headache. At the time of study enrollment, there was no standard definition of migraine, and thus multiple headache types may have been included in the study. In addition, only those who completed the study were included in the statistical analysis. In this study, 54% of placebo-treated patients dropped out, compared to 48% of amitriptyline-treated groups. Although this difference was not statistically significant, it may still have introduced bias. Moreover, it is unclear if the study was powered to detect differences in subgroup analyses, and no statistical adjustments were made for multiple comparisons over time. This study is still the largest placebo-controlled trial of amitriptyline vs. placebo, and despite its many limitations, it found a positive effect of amitriptyline prophylaxis for individuals with frequent migraines. In clinical practice, amitriptyline remains first-line for prophylaxis in individuals with both chronic daily headache and intermittent headaches.

Question

Is amitriptyline a safe and effective therapy for the prevention of migraine headaches?

Answer

Yes, this large trial showed that amitriptyline of up to 100 mg/day can reduce frequency of migraine headaches in individuals who suffer from frequent migraines.

CHAPTER 89

DIVALPROEX FOR MIGRAINE PROPHYLAXIS

Migraine Prophylaxis with Divalproex

Mathew NT, Saper JR, Silberstein SD, et al. *Arch Neurol*. 1995;52(3):281–286

BACKGROUND

This was the first study to demonstrate the effectiveness of divalproex for the prevention of migraine headaches. Prior to this study, several small open-label studies of valproate showed promising results for multiple types of headaches (persistent chronic daily headache, cluster headaches, and migraine headaches), which prompted this large multicenter trial.

OBJECTIVES

To evaluate the safety and efficacy of divalproex for migraine prophylaxis.

METHODS

Randomized, placebo-controlled, double-blind, parallel-group clinical trial of 107 patients enrolled across eight different neurology clinics throughout the United States.

Patients

Patients were individuals aged 16 to 75 (76% female, 94.5% white) who met International Headache Society Criteria for a diagnosis of migraine with or without aura for at least 6 months, and who had a migraine frequency of at least two episodes per month for 3 months. Notable exclusion criteria included women of childbearing potential, headaches more than 15 times a month, cluster headaches, significant medical or psychiatric disorders, poor medication compliance, prior valproate use, use of other migraine prophylactic medication, and daily use of analgesics such as ergotamines or NSAIDs.

Interventions

During the 4-week baseline phase, patients took daily placebo tablets and recorded headache frequency, severity, and duration. Patients who had two or more migraines during the baseline period, and were compliant with the headache diary, then progressed to the treatment phase (12 weeks). Patients were randomized in a 2:1 ratio of divalproex to placebo. Patients who were assigned the divalproex arm received 250 mg daily and increased the dose every 2 to 3 days until serum levels reached 70 to 120 mg/L, with a goal of 750 mg daily total dosing.

Outcomes

The primary endpoint was 4-week migraine headache frequency during the treatment phase. Secondary endpoints included (1) proportion of patients with 50% or more reduction in 4-week migraine headache frequency compared to baseline phase, (2) average duration of migraines, (3) average severity of migraine headache at peak intensity (peak severity), (4) assessment of functional restriction, and (5) average number of days per month headache "rescue" medications were used.

KEY RESULTS

- Divalproex group had a significantly lower monthly mean headache frequency compared to placebo group (3.5 vs. 5.7, $p < 0.001$) during the treatment phase.
- A significantly higher proportion of patients who received divalproex showed a 50% or more reduction in headache frequency, compared to patients receiving placebo (48% vs. 14%, $p < 0.001$).
- Divalproex-treated patients had significantly less functional restriction and used significantly less migraine-rescue medication per headache episode compared to placebo-treated patients.
- There was no significant change in headache duration or severity.
- Average dose of divalproex was 1,087 mg/day, reached in a mean of 13.4 days. Mean valproate sodium trough concentration was 66 mg/L.
- The use of divalproex was associated with nausea, somnolence, fatigue, vomiting, tremor, and alopecia. Side effects most often occurred during the dose titration period of the study, and 13% of patients treated with divalproex withdrew because of drug intolerance compared to 5% in placebo group (not statistically significant).

STUDY CONCLUSIONS

Divalproex is a generally well-tolerated, effective prophylactic therapy for migraine headaches.

COMMENTARY

This study provided strong evidence that valproate reduced the frequency of migraine headaches. Similar to results from other migraine-preventative medication trials, divalproex did not reduce the severity or duration of headaches when compared to placebo; however, it did reduce headache frequency, improve quality of life, and decrease the amount of migraine rescue medication that was required on a monthly basis. Although this study targeted a valproate level of 70 to 120 mg/L, this study did not show that a serum valproate level of 70 to 120 mg/L was necessary for efficacy. Currently, there is no evidence that a therapeutic serum valproate level is more effective than a subtherapeutic level in migraine prophylaxis; indeed, a 2001 study[1] showed that lower serum levels of valproate may even be more effective in migraine prevention than therapeutic levels. Of note, patient population was primarily white females without any significant medical or psychiatric comorbidities, and who took no other migraine preventative medications. This study was funded in part by Abbott Laboratories, the company that manufactures Depakote and other trade name formulations of divalproex.

Question

Is divalproex a safe and effective treatment for prevention of migraine headaches?

Answer

Yes. Because patients may experience benefit with subtherapeutic levels of valproate, dosing should be based on clinical response rather than therapeutic level.

Reference

1. Kinze S, Clauss M, Reuter U, et al. Valproic acid is effective in migraine prophylaxis at low serum levels: a prospective open-label study. *Headache.* 2001;41(8):774–778.

Scott M. McGinnis ■ Emer McGrath

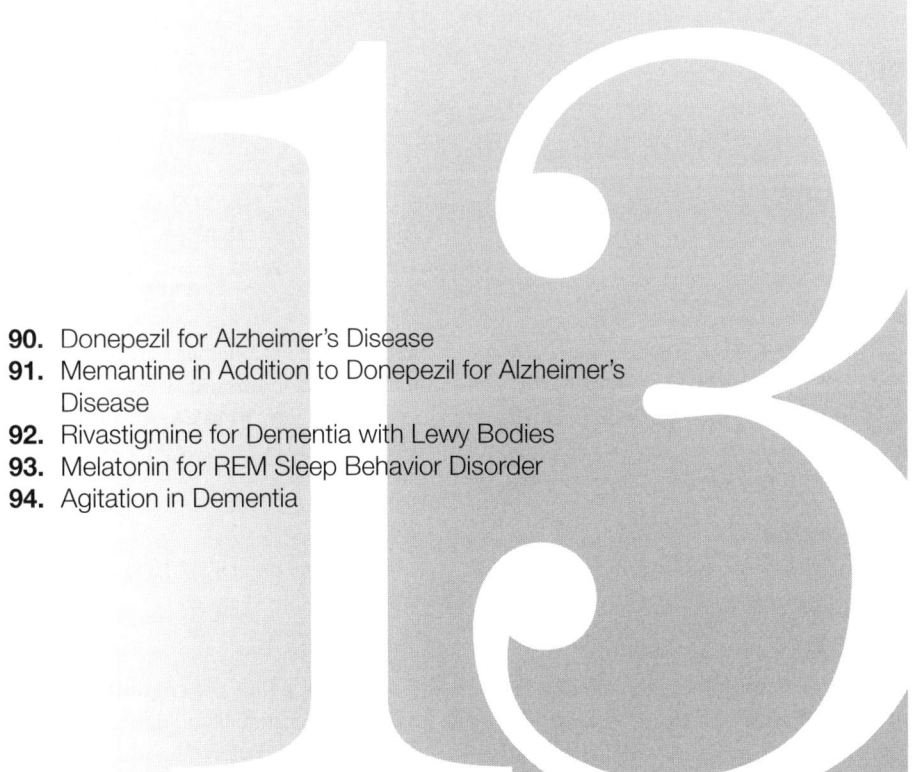

CHAPTER 90

DONEPEZIL FOR ALZHEIMER'S DISEASE

A 24-Week, Double-Blind, Placebo-Controlled Trial of Donepezil in Patients with Alzheimer's Disease

Rogers SL, Farlow MR, Doody RS, et al. *Neurology*. 1998;50:136–145

BACKGROUND

In patients with Alzheimer's disease (AD), memory and cognitive deficits have been associated with reduced presynaptic cholinergic function. Use of cholinergic agents may improve memory and cognitive symptoms in these patients. Donepezil, a cholinesterase inhibitor with relatively little peripheral anticholinesterase activity and a longer duration of action, offers advantages compared to less selective cholinesterase inhibitors. Prior to this study, there were no prior phase III RCTs evaluating the efficacy and safety of donepezil in patients with mild-to-moderate AD dementia.

OBJECTIVES

To evaluate the efficacy and safety of donepezil compared to placebo in patients with mild-to-moderate AD dementia.

METHODS

A randomized, double-blinded, placebo-controlled, parallel-group phase III trial at 20 US sites.

Patients

473 patients aged ≥50 years with a diagnosis of probable AD dementia according to National Institute of Neurological and Communicative Disorders and Alzheimer's Disease and Related Disorders Association criteria, MMSE score 10 to 26 (mean 19), and Clinical Dementia Rating (CDR) global score of 1 to 2 (indicating mild-to-moderate dementia) were enrolled.

Interventions

Participants were randomized to receive donepezil 5 mg/day ($n = 154$), donepezil 10 mg/day ($n = 157$), or placebo ($n = 162$) for 24 weeks.

Outcomes

Primary outcomes included change from baseline to week 24 on the cognitive portion of the Alzheimer's Disease Assessment Scale (ADAS-cog; range 0 to 70, higher scores indicate greater cognitive impairment) and the Clinician's Interview-Based Impression of Change-Plus (CIBIC-plus, a global function score derived from a structured clinical interview/examination with patient and caregiver; range 1 to 7: score of 1 indicates marked improvement, 4 indicates no change, and 7 indicates marked worsening). Secondary outcomes included MMSE (range 0 to 30, higher score indicates better cognitive function), the CDR-Sum of the Boxes scale (Clinical Dementia Rating Scale Sum of Boxes [CDR-SB], a consensus-based global clinical measure), and patient-rated Quality of Life (QoL) scale (7-item scale).

KEY RESULTS
- Compared to placebo, treatment with donepezil 5 mg/day and 10 mg/day resulted in a more favorable mean change in ADAS-cog scores from baseline to study endpoint (1.82 vs. -0.67, difference -2.49, $p < 0.0001$) and (1.82 vs. -1.06, difference -2.88, $p < 0.0001$), respectively. In addition, compared to placebo, treatment with donepezil 5 mg/day and 10 mg/day resulted in a more favorable mean change in CIBIC-plus scores from baseline to study endpoint (-0.97 vs. 0.24, difference 1.21, $p < 0.0007$) and (-0.97 vs. 0.39 difference 1.36, $p < 0.0002$), respectively.
- At the end of the 6-week placebo washout phase, ADAS-cog scores and CIBIC-plus ratings were not significantly different for the three groups
- There were also significant treatment benefits in both the 5 mg/day and 10 mg/day donepezil groups for the MMSE and CDR-SB, but not for patient-related QoL.
- Treatment discontinuation because of adverse events occurred in 7% of patients receiving placebo, 6% of patients receiving donepezil, and 16% of patients receiving donepezil 10 mg/day, largely due to gastrointestinal anticholinergic effects (diarrhea, nausea, and vomiting).

STUDY CONCLUSIONS
In patients, with mild-to-moderate AD dementia, donepezil results in improved cognitive and global function compared to placebo, and it is well tolerated.

COMMENTARY

This was the first phase III RCT to evaluate the efficacy and safety of donepezil in patients with mild-to-moderate AD dementia. Based on the results of this trial, the use of donepezil in patients with mild-to-moderate AD dementia was supported. Since the study, additional trials have supported the use of galantamine and rivastigmine, cholinesterase inhibitors similar to donepezil. Important caveats: this study did not include patients with mild cognitive impairment or vascular dementia, and so results from this trial cannot be generalized to these populations. Patients with greater comorbidities or those using concomitant antidepressant or antipsychotic medications were excluded, thus limiting the generalizability of results to patients at higher risk of poor medication tolerability or medication interactions.

Question
In patients with mild-to-moderate AD dementia, does donepezil result in improved outcomes compared to placebo?

Answer
Yes, donepezil results in improved cognitive and functional outcomes in patients with mild-to-moderate AD dementia, as observed in comparison to placebo after 12, 18, and 24 weeks.

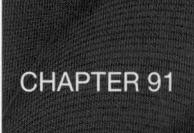

MEMANTINE IN ADDITION TO DONEPEZIL FOR ALZHEIMER'S DISEASE

CHAPTER 91

Memantine Treatment in Patients with Moderate-to-Severe Alzheimer's Disease Already Receiving Donepezil: A Randomized Controlled Trial

Tariot PN, Farlow MR, Grossberg GT, et al. *JAMA*. 2004;291(3):317–324

BACKGROUND

Glutamate is the primary excitatory neurotransmitter in the CNS. The NMDA receptor, which is activated by glutamate, is involved in learning and memory. Excessive NMDA stimulation by glutamate is thought to contribute to the pathogenesis of AD through excitotoxicty and neuronal cell death. Memantine is a noncompetitive NMDA receptor antagonist and may protect against further damage in AD dementia. Prior to this study, RCTs had demonstrated the safety and efficacy of memantine monotherapy for patients with moderate-to-severe AD dementia; however, no trials had evaluated the efficacy of memantine, in addition to a cholinesterase inhibitor, in patients with moderate-to-severe AD dementia.

OBJECTIVES

To compare the efficacy and safety of memantine vs. placebo in patients with moderate-to-severe AD dementia already receiving a stable treatment with donepezil.

METHODS

A randomized, double-blinded, placebo-controlled, parallel-group trial at 37 US sites.

Patients

404 patients aged ≥50 years with a diagnosis of probable AD according to National Institute of Neurological and Communicative Disorders and Stroke–Alzheimer's Disease and Related Disorders Association criteria, Mini-Mental State Examination score 5 to 14 (mean 10), MRI or CT scan within previous 12 months consistent with a diagnosis of probable AD, and cholinesterase inhibitor therapy with donepezil for >6 months before trial enrolment and at a stable dose (5 to 10 mg/day) for ≥3 months were enrolled between June 2001 and June 2002.

Interventions

Participants were randomized to receive memantine (starting dose 5 mg/day, increased to 20 mg/day, $n = 203$) or placebo ($n = 201$) for 24 weeks. Drug and placebo tablets were visually identical. A 1- to 2-week single-blind placebo run-in phase was completed prior to randomization to assess compliance.

Outcomes

Primary outcomes included change from baseline to week 24 on the Severe Impairment Battery (SIB) cognitive test (range 0 to 100) and on a modified 19-item Alzheimer's

Disease Cooperative Study–Activities of Daily Living Inventory (ADCS-ADL19, range 0 to 54). Higher scores indicated better function for both. Secondary outcomes included a Clinician's Interview-Based Impression of Change Plus Caregiver Input (CIBIC-Plus, used to assess effect of medication on clinical status; range 1 to 7: low scores indicated marked improvement, high scores indicated marked worsening), the Neuropsychiatric Inventory (NPI; range 0 to 144: higher score indicated worse symptoms), and the Behavioral Rating Scale for Geriatric Patients (BGP Care Dependency Subscale; range 0 to 70: higher score indicated worse function).

KEY RESULTS

- Combination memantine and donepezil, compared to placebo and donepezil, resulted in more favorable changes in total mean scores on the SIB (0.9 vs. -2.5, $p < 0.001$) and ASCS-ADL19 (-2.0 vs. -3.4, $p = 0.03$) inventories, respectively.
- Combination therapy, compared to placebo, resulted in more favorable total mean CIBIC-Plus scores (4.41 vs. 4.66, respectively, $p = 0.03$), as well as more favorable changes in total mean scores on the NPI (-0.1 vs. 3.7, $p = 0.002$) and BGP (0.8 vs. 2.3, $p = 0.001$)
- Treatment discontinuation because of adverse events occurred in 7.4% of patients randomized to memantine compared to 12.4% randomized to placebo.

STUDY CONCLUSIONS

In patients with moderate-to-severe AD dementia receiving stable doses of donepezil, memantine resulted in significantly better outcomes than placebo on measures of cognition, activities of daily living, global outcome, and behavior and was well tolerated.

COMMENTARY

In 2001, the only FDA-approved treatment for AD dementia was a cholinesterase inhibitor. This was the first randomized, double-blinded, placebo-controlled trial to show a benefit of memantine, in addition to cholinesterase inhibitor therapy, in patients with moderate-to-severe AD dementia. Based on the results of this trial, the use of memantine in combination with a cholinesterase inhibitor in patients with advanced AD dementia was supported. Important caveats: This study did not include patients with vascular dementia, and so results from this trial cannot be generalized to this population. Only patients who were on stable long-term donepezil dosing were included; patients with greater comorbidities, and thus a greater risk of poor tolerability or medication interactions, were less likely to be included.

Question

In patients with moderate-to-severe AD dementia already receiving donepezil, is memantine more effective than placebo?

Answer

Yes, memantine, in addition to cholinesterase inhibitors, results in a small improvement in outcomes in patients with moderate-to-severe AD dementia.

CHAPTER 92

RIVASTIGMINE FOR DEMENTIA WITH LEWY BODIES

Efficacy of Rivastigmine in Dementia with Lewy Bodies: A Randomized, Double-Blind, Placebo-Controlled International Study

McKeith I, Del Ser T, PierFranco S, et al. *Lancet*. 2000;356:2031–2036

BACKGROUND

Reduced cholinergic function has been noted in patients with dementia with Lewy bodies (DLB). Drugs that enhance cholinergic function, such as the cholinesterase inhibitor rivastigmine, may offer a therapeutic option for patients with DLB. Prior to this study, there were no prior randomized, blinded, controlled trials evaluating the efficacy and safety of rivastigmine in patients with probable DLB.

OBJECTIVES

To compare the efficacy and safety of donepezil vs. placebo in patients with probable DLB.

METHODS

A randomized, double-blinded, placebo-controlled, parallel-group trial at sites in Spain, United Kingdom, and Italy.

Patients

120 patients with a clinical diagnosis of probable DLB and mild-to-moderate dementia as defined by an MMSE score above 9 were enrolled. Patients with severe extrapyramidal symptoms, defined as a Hoehn and Yahr score over 3, or scores over 3 for rigidity, tremor, or bradykinesia on the Unified Parkinson's Disease Rating Scale (UPDRS), and those who were on neuroleptics, anticholinergics, selegiline, or similar drugs, were not included.

Interventions

Participants were randomized to receive rivastigmine (starting dose 1.5 mg twice a day, increased to 6 mg twice a day, $n = 59$) or placebo ($n = 61$) for 20 weeks. Drug and placebo tablets were visually identical.

Outcomes

Primary outcomes included a neuropsychiatric inventory 4 (NPI-4) subscore (a four-item subscore calculated as the sum of scores for delusions, hallucinations, apathy, and depression, previously identified as the main Lewy-body dementia cluster) and a combined score indicating the speed of response to selected tests from the cognitive drug research computerized cognitive assessment system (tests attention, working memory, and episodic memory). Secondary outcomes included the clinical global change-plus (CGC-plus); the total score of NPI items one to ten (NPI-10); the MMSE; and other combined scores from the computerized cognitive assessment tests, the individual tasks, and additional neuropsychological tests for executive function and planning (digit symbol substitution task, trail-making tests A and B, controlled word association test, Stroop test, and block-design test).

KEY RESULTS

- There was no difference in the mean change in NPI-4 scores from baseline to follow-up between donepezil and placebo groups in the intention to treat dataset. However, in the last observation carried forward dataset, donepezil, compared to placebo, resulted in more favorable changes in total mean NPI-4 (3.1 vs. 0.8 $p = 0.045$) and NPI-10 (5.0 vs. 1.2, $p = 0.048$) scores.
- In the computerized cognitive assessment system speed score, patients receiving rivastigmine were faster and better than those on placebo, particularly on tasks with a substantial attentional component ($p = 0.048$ for intent to treat dataset, $p = 0.046$ in last observation carried forward dataset).
- There was no significant difference in the mean change in CGC-plus or MMSE scores between rivastigmine or placebo groups over 20 weeks.
- Patients taking rivastigmine showed significantly less anxiety, delusions and hallucinations compared to controls.
- After drug discontinuation for 3 weeks, the mean differences between trial arms were no longer significant.
- A higher proportion of patients randomized to rivastigmine compared to placebo experienced adverse events (predominantly cholinergic gastrointestinal adverse events): 92% vs. 75%, respectively.

STUDY CONCLUSIONS

Rivastigmine 6 to 12 mg daily produces statistically and clinically significant behavioral effects in patients with Lewy-body dementia, and it seems safe and well tolerated if titrated individually.

COMMENTARY

Prior to this study, there were no randomized, blinded, controlled trials evaluating the efficacy and safety of rivastigmine in patients with probable DLB. This study provides evidence to support the use of rivastigmine in patients with DLB. Important caveats: This study did not include patients with severe dementia or those with severe extrapyramidal symptoms, thus results from this trial cannot be generalized to this population. Only 69% of patients assigned to rivastigmine and 84% assigned to placebo completed the study. Many patients in the rivastigmine group prematurely discontinued the study drug because of intolerance.

Question

In patients with probable DLB, is rivastigmine more effective than placebo in improving neuropsychiatric symptoms?

Answer

Yes, rivastigmine results in improved neuropsychiatric function in patients with probable DLB.

CHAPTER 93

MELATONIN FOR REM SLEEP BEHAVIOR DISORDER

Melatonin for Treatment of REM Sleep Behavior Disorder in Neurologic Disorders: Results in 14 Patients

Boeve BF, Silber MH, Ferman TJ. *Sleep Med.* 2003;4:281–284

BACKGROUND

Rapid eye movement (REM) sleep behavior disorder (RBD) is characterized by loss of normal skeletal muscle atonia during REM sleep with prominent motor activity and disturbed dreaming. Clonazepam has previously been considered the treatment of choice for RBD. In patients with symptoms refractory to clonazepam or who are unable to tolerate clonazepam, there are no good treatment alternatives. Melatonin has been proposed as a potential alternative to clonazepam based on the results of an open-label trial. However, to date, there have been minimal published data and limited follow-up on the use of melatonin in patients with RBD.

OBJECTIVES

To describe the treatment response with melatonin for RBD associated with other neurologic disorders.

METHODS

A retrospective analysis of clinical records for consecutive patients with RBD treated with melatonin at the Mayo Clinic between 2001 and 2002.

Patients

14 consecutive patients (median age 56, range 20 to 77years) with a diagnosis of RBD who were experiencing dream enactment behavior one or more nights per week and in whom some form of treatment was considered clinically necessary because of potentially injurious behavior.

Interventions

Patients were started on over-the-counter melatonin at 3 mg/night, increased in 3 mg increments to a maximum of 12 mg/night every five to seven nights as necessary and tolerated.

Outcomes

The primary outcome was patient's and bed partner's self-reported melatonin response, categorized as one of the following: RBD controlled, RBD markedly improved but not eliminated, RBD initially improved but subsequently returned, RBD not significantly changed, or RBD worsened. The mean duration of follow-up was 14 months (range 9 to 25)

KEY RESULTS

- RBD was controlled in six patients, significantly improved in four, and RBD initially improved but subsequently returned in two. No improvement occurred in one patient. Increased RBD frequency and severity occurred in one patient.
- The effective melatonin doses were 3 mg in two cases, 6 mg in seven cases, 9 mg in one case, and 12 mg in two cases.
- Five patients reported side effects which resolved with decreased dosage, including morning headaches (2), morning sleepiness (2), and delusions/hallucinations (1).
- Eight patients experienced continued benefit with melatonin beyond 12 months of therapy.

STUDY CONCLUSIONS

Melatonin can be considered as a possible sole or add-on therapy in select patients with RBD. Prospective, long-term, controlled trials with melatonin are warranted in a larger number of patients with RBD associated with a variety of neurologic symptoms and disorders.

COMMENTARY

Clonazepam has previously been considered the treatment of choice for RBD. However, in patients with symptoms refractory to clonazepam or who are unable to tolerate clonazepam, there are no good treatment alternatives. This issue arises frequently in populations with dementia with Lewy bodies and Parkinson disease dementia—synucleinopathies with high prevalence of RBD and risk of exacerbation of cognitive and neuropsychiatric symptoms with benzodiazepines. This retrospective analysis aimed to describe the treatment response with melatonin for patients with RBD and provides low-quality evidence to potentially support the use of melatonin as a second-line agent to clonazepam in patients with RBD. Important caveats: This was not a prospective, randomized, blinded trial. In addition, there was no control group available for comparison, thus the efficacy of melatonin for RBD cannot be determined from this study. The results are confounded by the continued use of clonazepam in seven patients in the setting of small sample size. Different over-the-counter formulations of melatonin were used in the study, which may have resulted in varying tolerability according to brand used. The outcome measure was subjective, based on patient's and bed partner's self-reported response, increasing the risk of reporting bias. Finally, the majority of patients were men, thus results may not be generalizable to women.

Question

In patients with RBD associated with other neurologic disorders, is melatonin associated with a favorable treatment response?

Answer

Yes, this study provides low-quality evidence to suggest that melatonin may be associated with a favorable treatment response in patients with RBD. However, before recommending this treatment, randomized, blinded controlled trials are required to evaluate the efficacy of melatonin for patients with RBD.

CHAPTER 94

AGITATION IN DEMENTIA

Nonpharmacological Interventions for Agitation in Dementia: Systematic Review of Randomized Controlled Trials

Livingston G, Kelly L, Lewis-Holmes E, et al. *Br J Psychiatry*. 2014;205:436–442

BACKGROUND

Agitation in dementia is common, persistent, distressing, and can lead to care breakdown. Medication is often ineffective and harmful, and it can result in increased cognitive decline. There has only been one published, well-conducted systematic review of nonpharmacological management of agitation in dementia to date. However, this review only included RCTs published before 2004, it did not consider the duration of the intervention effect or whether the intervention was preventive or treated clinically significant agitation.

OBJECTIVES

To systematically review the evidence for nonpharmacological interventions for agitation in people with dementia.

METHODS

A systematic review and qualitative synthesis of RCTs ($n > 45$) of nonpharmacological interventions for agitation in patients with dementia. Papers were rated for quality, using the Centre for Evidence-Based Medicine (CEBM) RCT evaluation criteria.

Patients

Patients with dementia. Studies in which participants were administered psychotropic drugs were excluded.

Interventions

Nonpharmacological interventions for agitation were included.

Outcomes

Agitation was defined as inappropriate verbal, vocal, or motor activity not judged by an outside observer to be an outcome of need, encompassing physical and verbal aggression and wandering. A score above 39 on the Cohen-Mansfield Agitation Inventory (CMAI) and a score above 4 on the NPI agitation scale indicated significant agitation.

KEY RESULTS

- Person-centered care, communication skills training, and adapted dementia care mapping decreased symptomatic and severe agitation in care homes immediately (standardized effect sizes [SES] range 0.3 to 1.8) and for up to 6 months afterwards (SES range 0.2 to 2.2). There was no evidence in other settings.

- Activities and music therapy by protocol (SES range 0.5 to 0.6) decreased overall agitation, while sensory intervention decreased clinically significant agitation immediately.
- Aromatherapy and light therapy did not demonstrate efficacy.

STUDY CONCLUSIONS

Interventions that emphasize communicating with dementia patients and helping staff to understand and fulfill the wishes of people with dementia can reduce both symptomatic and severe agitation during the intervention as well as 3 to 6 months afterwards.

COMMENTARY

Medication is often ineffective and harmful for management of agitation in patients with dementia. There have been no recent systematic reviews of nonpharmacological management of agitation in dementia that have considered the duration of the intervention effect or whether the intervention was effective in preventing or treating clinically significant agitation. In this systematic review among patients with dementia living in care homes, person-centered care, communication skills training, and adapted dementia care mapping decreased symptomatic and severe agitation immediately and up to 6 months afterwards. Benefits were also noted with activities therapy and music therapy, though with smaller effect sizes. Caveats include: this review is subject to publication bias because of the higher proportion of negative trials that are not published. Given the significant heterogeneity in the intervention and method of measuring agitation between trials, it was not possible to complete a meta-analysis to quantitatively measure a treatment effect. Many of the included studies were also underpowered to detect a treatment effect.

Question

In patients with dementia and agitation, is there evidence to support the use of nonpharmacological interventions for agitation?

Answer

Yes, this review provides evidence to support the use of nonpharmacological interventions, namely, person-centered care and communication skills training, for the short- and long-term management of agitation in patients with dementia.

SECTION 14

PEDIATRIC NEUROLOGY

Patricia L. Musolino ■ Melissa A. Walker

CHAPTER 95

TREATMENT OF INFANTILE SPASMS

The United Kingdom Infantile Spasms Study (UKISS) Comparing Hormone Treatment with Vigabatrin on Developmental and Epilepsy Outcomes to Age 14 Months: A Multicentre Randomised Trial

Lux AL, Edwards SW, Hancock E, et al. *Lancet Neurol.* 2005;4(11):712–717

BACKGROUND

Prior to 2005, observational trials and clinical experience suggested that patients with infantile spasms (IS) who responded to therapy with cessation of spasms might have improved developmental outcomes; but this hypothesis had not been tested in a prospective manner. In a previously published article, a cohort of infants with IS (United Kingdom Infantile Spasms Study, UKISS) were randomized to either hormone therapy (prednisolone or synthetic adrenocorticotropic hormone) or vigabatrin and followed for cessation of spasms after 14 days of treatment. The authors reported a higher response rate in patients receiving hormonal therapy.[1]

OBJECTIVES

To assess developmental outcomes in patients with cessation of spasms compared to those who did not— comparison by treatment, time until treatment, and etiology of IS.

METHODS

Prospective observational study at 150 hospitals in the United Kingdom.

Patients

107 patients aged 2 to 12 months with IS, originally randomized to either hormonal or vigabatrin therapy and followed for cessation of spasms as reported in 2004.[1] Exclusion criteria included diagnosis of or "high risk of" tuberous sclerosis, previous IS treatment within the past 28 days, contraindications to hormone or vigabatrin treatment, or second potentially lethal disorder.

Interventions

Treatment of IS with either hormone therapy or vigabatrin was undertaken as previously published.[1]

Outcomes

Developmental assessments were performed using the Vineland Adaptive Behavioral Scales (VABS) by phone at 14 months of age.

KEY RESULTS

- VABS scores were obtained for 101 of 102 surviving patients.
- No significant difference in composite scores was observed between the cohort treated with hormone therapy and the cohort treated with vigabatrin (78.6 [SD = 16.8] vs. 77.5 [12.7], difference 1.0, 95% CI, 4.9 to 7.0, $t_{99} = 0.35$, $p = 0.73$).

- No significant difference was observed between patients who started treatment within 1 month and those who started after 1 month (80.3 [14.9] vs. 76.1 [15.1], difference 4.3, 95% CI, 2.2 to 10.7, $t_{89} = 1.32, p = 0.19$).
- Mean composite scores were significantly higher in patients with cryptogenic IS compared to those with an identified, symptomatic etiology (83.8 [16.5] vs. 73.3 [11.4], difference 10.5, 95% CI, 4.9 to 16.1, $t_{97} = 3.74, p = 0.0003$).
- In patients with cryptogenic IS, mean composite scores were higher in patients treated with hormone therapy compared to vigabatrin (88.2 [17.3] vs. 78.9 [14.3], difference 9.3, 95% CI, 1.2 to 17.3, least significant difference test, $t_{95} = 2.28, p = 0.025$).

STUDY CONCLUSIONS

Patients who respond to treatment have better developmental outcomes than patients who do not. Patients with cryptogenic IS have better developmental outcomes than those with symptomatic etiologies. There is no significant difference in developmental outcomes between patients treated with hormonal therapy and those treated with vigabatrin, with the exception of patients with cryptogenic IS, who may experience better developmental outcomes when treated with hormonal therapy.

COMMENTARY

Although causation cannot be proven, the results presented by this study support treatment of IS with either hormonal or vigabatrin with the goal of improving developmental outcomes, a concept well supported within the field. It is unlikely that definitive proof that treatment results in improved developmental outcomes will ever be obtained given the ethical dilemmas inherent in conducting such a trial. To date, the selection of initial therapy (prednisolone vs. adrenocorticotropic hormone vs. vigabatrin) remains controversial, with perhaps the limited exception of a sole etiologic subset (tuberous sclerosis), particularly given that these therapies vary significantly in cost and associated morbidities. As our understanding of the multiple etiologies of IS deepens, it is likely that additional etiology-specific regimens, protocols, and prognostication will be available to patients.

Question

Is cessation of IS in the setting of medical treatment associated with improved developmental outcomes?

Answer

Yes.

Reference

1. Lux AL, Edwards SW, Hancock E, et al. The United Kingdom Infantile Spasms Study comparing vigabatrin with prednisolone or tetracosactide at 14 days: a multicentre, randomised controlled trial. *Lancet.* 2004;364(9447):1773–1778.

CHAPTER 96

PHARMACO VS. BEHAVIORAL THERAPY FOR ADHD

A 14-Month Randomized Clinical Trial of Treatment Strategies for Attention-Deficit/Hyperactivity Disorder. The MTA Cooperative Group. Multimodal Treatment Study of Children with ADHD

The MTA Cooperative Group. *Arch Gen Psychiatry*. 1999;56(12):1073–1086

BACKGROUND

Prior to 1999, there were no long-term (>3 months) controlled studies of socio-demographically diverse cohorts comparing medical and behavioral therapies for attention-deficit/hyperactivity disorder (ADHD) that were of size sufficient to identify statistically significant predictors of treatment response.

OBJECTIVES

To compare long-term medical, behavioral, and combined medical and behavioral ADHD therapies relative to each other and to routine community care.

METHODS

Prospective randomized, controlled study at six centers across the United States.

Patients

579 children with ADHD Combined Type, aged 7 to 9.9 years, were randomized to 14 months of medication management, intensive behavioral treatment, combined medication and intensive behavioral management, or standard community care. Exclusions included history of chronic tics or Tourette syndrome, bipolar disorder, psychosis, personality disorder, Weschler Intelligence Scale for Children score of <80, major neurologic or medical illness, and/or non-English-speaking primary caretaker, among others.

Interventions

Children received 14 months of medication management (methylphenidate therapy), intensive behavioral treatment, combined medication and intensive behavioral management, or standard community care.

Outcomes
- Impulsivity SNAP (acronym denoting the developers' names) rating subscale completed by parents and teachers.
- Oppositional-defiant SNAP rating subscale completed by parents and teachers.
- Social skills rating system (SSRS) social skill subscale rating by parents and teachers.
- SSRS internalizing (anxiety and depression) subscale ratings by parents and teachers.
- Parent–child relationship questionnaire.
- Wechsler Individual Achievement Test subscales (reading, math, and spelling) for academic achievement.

KEY RESULTS

- Medical therapy showed superior efficacy to behavioral therapy in parents' and teachers' ratings of inattention and teachers' ratings of hyperactivity/impulsivity; there were no differences in any other domains between the two groups.
- Combined treatment was superior to behavioral therapy alone per parents' and teachers' ratings of inattention, parents' ratings of hyperactivity/impulsivity, parents' SNAP oppositional/aggressive subscales, and Weschler Individual Achievement Test reading scores.
- Medical or combined therapies showed significant benefit compared to community care in all ADHD symptom domains whereas behavioral therapy did not.

STUDY CONCLUSIONS

Medical therapy (methylphenidate) is superior to behavioral therapy for treatment of ADHD symptoms. Combined medical and behavioral therapy shows no additional benefit for ADHD symptoms, but may improve non-ADHD symptoms.

COMMENTARY

This study was designed to compare the benefits of long-term medical (methylphenidate), behavioral, and combined medical and behavioral therapies for the treatment of ADHD and related symptoms. Trepidation existed at the time regarding the long-term use of stimulants, and this study supported the use of long-term stimulant therapy using a large cohort and multiple assessment parameters provided by parents as well as teachers. Importantly, patients with tics were excluded and hesitations regarding the use of stimulants persist to date, despite meta-analysis of several trials suggesting that psychostimulants do not increase the risk of tics.[1]

Question

Is medical, behavioral, or combined therapy more efficacious for the treatment of ADHD?

Answer

Medical therapy is the most efficacious treatment for symptoms of ADHD.

Reference

1. Millichap JG. Risk of Tics with psychostimulants for ADHD. *Pediatr Neurol Briefs.* 2015;29(12):95.

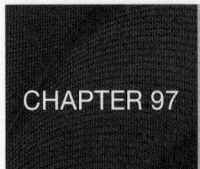

CHAPTER 97

KETOGENIC DIET FOR THE TREATMENT OF CHILDHOOD EPILEPSY

The Ketogenic Diet for the Treatment of Childhood Epilepsy: A Randomized Controlled Trial

Neal EG, Chaffe H, Schwartz RH, et al. *Lancet Neurol*. 2008;7:500–506

BACKGROUND

Improved seizure control under circumstances inducing ketonemia date to the 1920s, but prior to this time, no RCTs had been undertaken to assess the efficacy of ketogenic diets in seizure control.

OBJECTIVES

To assess the efficacy of ketogenic diet for seizure control in children with epilepsy.

METHODS

Prospective, randomized, controlled multicenter trial in the United Kingdom.

Patients

145 children (aged 2 to 16 years) with seizures occurring ≥ 1 time daily or with ≥ 7 seizures/week refractory to ≥ 2 AEDs not previously treated with ketogenic diet. Exclusion criteria included history of hyperlipidemia, nephroliathisis, or organic acid deficiency syndrome. Patients with multiple seizure semiologies and epilepsy syndromes were included.

Interventions

Children were randomized to receive the ketogenic diet immediately or after a 3-month delay, or to no changes in current treatment. Diet tolerability was assessed by a questionnaire at 3 months.

Outcomes

Primary endpoint was reduction in seizures by intention to treat analysis.

KEY RESULTS

- Mean percentage of baseline seizures was significantly lower in diet-treated children compared to controls after 3 months (62.0% vs. 136.9%, 75% decrease, 95% CI, 42.2 to 107.4%, $p < 0.0001$).
- 28 children (38%) treated with diet experienced >50% reduction in seizures compared with 4 controls (6%) after 3 months ($p < 0.0001$).
- 5 children treated with diet experienced >90% seizure reduction compared with no controls after 3 months ($p = 0.00582$).

STUDY CONCLUSIONS

Ketogenic diet represents an effective treatment for refractory epilepsy in children.

COMMENTARY
This study was designed to validate a long-standing observation that ketogenesis increases the seizure threshold. Large-scale implementation of ketogenic diet following this and other studies has provided an important nonsurgical option for the management of epilepsy refractory to ≥2 AEDs in the pediatric population. Notably, a similar RCT of ketogenic diet for the treatment of refractory epilepsy in adults has yet to be completed.

Question

Is the ketogenic diet effective in treating refractory epilepsy in children?

Answer

Yes.

CHAPTER 98

HYPOTHERMIA FOR NEONATES WITH HYPOXIC-ISCHEMIC ENCEPHALOPATHY

Effects of Hypothermia for Perinatal Asphyxia on Childhood Outcomes

Azzopardi D, Strohm B, Marlow N, et al. *NEJM*. 2014;371(2):140–149

BACKGROUND

Previous work in RCTs including the Total Body Hypothermia for Neonatal Encephalopathy Trial (TOBY) had demonstrated reduced risk of death or disability at 18 to 24 months of age and increased likelihood of survival without disability in infants demonstrating clear evidence of asphyxia encephalopathy treated with therapeutic hypothermia compared to controls.[1] No assessment at a later time point had yet been reported in patients who received this therapeutic hypothermia.

OBJECTIVES

To assess neurocognitive function of individuals receiving therapeutic hypothermia compared to controls at age 6 to 7 years.

METHODS

Prospective randomized, controlled multicenter study.

Patients

277 patients born at a gestational age $\geq$ 36 weeks with clear evidence of asphyxia encephalopathy.

Interventions

Patients randomized to either moderate hypothermia (33°C to 34°C) or standard care for 72 hours initiated within 6 hours of birth. Evaluations included neurologic examination, psychometric assessment with Wechsler Preschool and Primary Scale of Intelligence (WPPSI-III) or Wechsler Intelligence Scale for Children IV (WISC-IV), and Neuropsychological Assessment II (NEPSY-II) subsets including attention and executive function, visuospatial processing, sensorimotor function, and memory and learning.

Outcomes

Frequency of survival with intelligence quotient (IQ) score $\geq$ 85 (1 standard deviation below the general population mean)

KEY RESULTS

- There was no statistically significant difference in survival at 6 to 7 years between treated and control groups (29% vs. 30%, respectively).
- There was no statistically significant difference in parental assessments of children health status between treated and control groups.

- 52% (75) children in the hypothermia group compared to 39% (52) in the control group survived with an IQ of $\geq$ 85 at age 6 to 7 years (relative risk 1.31, $p = 0.04$).
- Abnormalities on neurologic exam were decreased in the treated group (65 patients, 45%) compared to controls (37 patients, 28%, relative risk 1.6, 95% CI, 1.15 to 2.22).
- The risk of cerebral palsy was reduced in the treated group (21%) compared to controls (36%, $p = 0.03$).
- There was no statistically significant difference between treated and control groups in psychometric tests with the exception of attention and executive function, where the control group scored lower on average than the treated group ($p = 0.03$).

STUDY CONCLUSIONS

Therapeutic hypothermia compared to standard treatment for infants with encephalopathy after birth asphyxia results in improved neurocognitive outcomes that are demonstrable in middle childhood.

COMMENTARY

This study was the first to investigate neurocognitive outcomes in patients treated with therapeutic hypothermia for encephalopathy after birth asphyxia in childhood. The results demonstrate lasting beneficial effects of therapy in surviving patients, validating the current status of therapeutic hypothermia as standard of care for infants of $\geq$ 36 gestational age with encephalopathy after birth asphyxia.

Question

Does therapeutic hypothermia for infants with encephalopathy after birth asphyxia improve long-term neurocognitive outcomes?

Answer

Yes.

Reference

1. Jacobs SE, Berg M, Hunt R, et al. Cooling for newborns with hypoxic ischemic encephalopathy. *Cochrane Database Syst Rev.* 2013;1:CD003311.

CHAPTER 99 · FEBRILE SEIZURES

Factors Prognostic of Unprovoked Seizures after Febrile Convulsions
Annegers JF, Hauser A, Shirts SB, et al. *NEJM.* 1987;316(9):493–498

BACKGROUND
It had been unknown how long the risk of unprovoked seizure after febrile seizure persisted, or if semiology (e.g., focal features) was prognostic. This study was the first to follow patients into adulthood and examine independent risk factors for future unprovoked seizures.

OBJECTIVES
To determine features associated with risk of future unprovoked seizures in children with prior febrile seizures.

METHODS
Population-based, prospective cohort study using data from a US city from 1935 to 1979.

Patients
687 children with febrile seizures without history of prior unprovoked seizure. Select exclusion criteria: IQ <70, cerebral palsy, and CNS infection.

Interventions
Demographic, clinical, and family data were collected for patients at the time of first febrile seizure. Medical records were then subsequently followed until occurrence of unprovoked seizure, out-of-area move, or until study end, for a total of >10,000 person-years (average 18 years/patient).

Outcomes
Primary outcome was development of unprovoked, afebrile seizures. Secondary outcomes were risk factors associated with subsequent seizure occurrence and seizure type.

KEY RESULTS
- Children with febrile seizures had an average 7% risk of later unprovoked seizures, with higher risk associated with focality (RR = 3.6, 95% CI, 1.4 to 9.1), duration >30 minutes (RR = 2.8, 95% CI, 1.0 to 7.8), and > 1 seizures in a 24-hour period (RR = 2.8, 95% CI, 1.3 to 6).
- Children experiencing simple febrile seizures had a 2.4% risk of unprovoked seizures through age 25 years, whereas those with complex features (but no other risk factors) had an 8% risk (95% CI, 3 to 19).

• Cumulative risk of unprovoked seizure increases with increasing number of complex features, with a 49% risk in children with focal features, repeated episodes, and prolonged duration.

STUDY CONCLUSIONS

In long-term follow-up, the absolute risk of subsequent unprovoked seizures in children with febrile seizures was low but increased with the presence of complex features.

COMMENTARY

Strengths of this study include its relatively large cohort size, the exclusive use of prospectively identified unprovoked seizures, and the inclusion of children born across a significant span of time. The single-city location as well as exclusion of patients retrospectively identified as having CNS infection, traumatic insult, low IQ, or cerebral palsy minimizes the impact of potentially important confounders. Finally, the study examines the risk of unprovoked seizure (single or multiple) as opposed to recurrent unprovoked seizures (epilepsy), which is the primary concern for most patients, families, and clinicians. Interestingly, a later, British national cohort study found that 6% of children with complex febrile seizures subsequently developed epilepsy.[1]

Question

What is the risk of subsequent unprovoked seizure in children with febrile seizures?

Answer

In general, there is a 7% overall risk of subsequent unprovoked seizure, but this risk varies from as low as 2% for simple febrile seizures to almost 50% for febrile seizures with multiple complex features.

Reference

1. Verity CM, Golding J. Risk of epilepsy after febrile convulsions: a national cohort study. *BMJ.* 1991;303(6814):1373–1376.

CHAPTER 100

WHEN TO STOP ANTIEPILEPTIC DRUGS IN CHILDREN WITH EPILEPSY

Recurrence Risk after Withdrawal of Antiepileptic Drugs in Children with Epilepsy: A Prospective Study

Ramos-Lizana J, Aguirre-Rodríguez J, Aguilera-Lopez P. *Eur J Paediatr Neurol.* 2010;14:116–124

BACKGROUND

Although it was known that children frequently outgrow epilepsy, previous studies provided little guidance on when an AED successfully used as monotherapy might be stopped with the lowest risk of recurrent seizure in the pediatric population. Therefore, this study analyzed remission after cessation of AEDs per current practice in a pediatric epilepsy cohort.

OBJECTIVES

To determine seizure recurrence risk and prognostic factors predicting relapse after AED withdrawal in children with epilepsy.

METHODS

Large, prospective, observational trial of children at a single center in Spain enrolled from 1994 to 2004.

Patients

353 children, aged 0 to 13 years, with a history of >2 unprovoked seizures separated by >24 hours. Select exclusion criteria: exclusive neonatal seizures, inborn error of metabolism, and neurodegenerative disorder.

Interventions

AED withdrawal after achieving epilepsy remission >2 years. Patients were then followed by in-person interview for 1 to 3 years and by telephone for at least 5 years. In addition, baseline and follow-up EEGs were obtained when possible. Some patients had baseline imaging.

Outcomes

Primary outcome was seizure recurrence risk after 2 years off AEDs.

KEY RESULTS

- 309/343 children were initially treated with AEDs. 238/309 children achieved remission (mean seizure-free time 2.16 ± 0.6 years), of which 216 consented to AED withdrawal.
- Seizure recurrence risk after AED withdrawal was 23% at 2 years (95% CI, 17 to 29) and 28% at 5 years (95% CI, 22 to 34).

- A significant increase in risk of seizure recurrence was noted with epilepsy secondary to an acquired insult (41%, 85% CI, 28 to 54), history of prior febrile seizures ($p < 0.05$), prior neonatal seizures ($p < 0.05$), global developmental delay ($p < 0.05$), abnormal neuroimaging ($p < 0.05$), and particular seizure types associated with epilepsy syndromes.

STUDY CONCLUSIONS

In children with epilepsy, recurrent seizure risk after withdrawal of AEDs is low. The etiology of an individual's epilepsy, particularly the presence of epilepsy associated with a known syndrome, is the primary predictor.

COMMENTARY

An earlier meta-analysis published with the practice parameters it informed described predictors of successful AED cessation as no seizures for 2 to 5 years, single type of partial or primary generalized tonic-clonic seizures, normal examination and normal IQ, and normalization of EEG on treatment.[1] In addition to the factors identified in this study, individual patient variables (including driving, activities/hobbies, and living situation) should be considered in the decision to attempt AED taper. Given the increased risk of seizure recurrence associated with particular syndromes and expansion of testing capabilities, future patient education will likely incorporate the results of genetics studies.

Question

Is it safe to consider stopping AEDs in children with epilepsy in remission?

Answer

Yes, if they have been seizure-free for 2 years and have specific low-risk epilepsy syndromes.

Reference

1. Practice parameter: a guideline for discontinuing antiepileptic drugs in seizure-free patients—summary statement. Report of the Quality Standards Subcommittee of the American Academy of Neurology. *Neurology*. 1996;47:600–602.

INDEX